AF522526

Rural Health

Rural Health
Perspectives and Experiences

Edited by
Azmal Hussain

2012

Icfai Books
The Icfai University Press

RURAL HEALTH: PERSPECTIVES AND EXPERIENCES

Editor: Azmal Hussain

First Edition: 2012
Printed in India

Published by

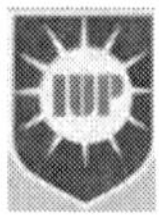

This book is published by IUP.
University Campus, Agartala-Simna Road,
P.O. Kamalghat Sadar, Agartala – 799210, Tripura (West)
E-mail: info@iupindia.org
Website: www.books.iupindia.org

ISBN: 978-81-314-2736-1

Contents

Overview I

SECTION I

DIMENSIONS

1. Rural Health: Current Dimensions 3
Azmal Hussain

2. Rural Health Insurance: A Hope for the Poor 16
Azmal Hussain

3. Chronic Disease Management Systems (Registries) in Rural Health Care 26
Anne Skinner, Roslyn Fraser-Maginn and Keith J Mueller

4. A Web-Based Graphical User Interface for Evidence-Based Decision-Making for Health Care Allocations in Rural Areas 37
Nadine Schuurman, Margo Leight and Myriam Berube

5. Bridging Rural Health Research and Policy: Dissemination Strategies 61
Keith J Mueller, Timothy D McBride, Andrew F Coburn, Rebecca T Slifkin, Mary K Wakefield and A Clinton MacKinney

SECTION II

PRACTICES

6. National Centre of Rural Medicine in Norway: A Bridge from Rural Practice to the Academy 73
IJ Aaraas and E Swensen

7. Quality through Collaboration: The Future of Rural & Frontier Emergency Medical Services in the US Health System 82
www.hrsa.gov

8. Rural Health Insurance – Rising to the Challenge 115
www-wds.worldbank.org

9. Telemedicine in Rural India 131
Sanjit Bagchi

10. Pre-Triage Procedures in Mobile Rural Health Clinics in Ethiopia 138
PC Stillman and PC Strong

11. Rural Community Well-Being: The Perspectives of Health Care Managers in Southwestern Manitoba, Canada 150
Doug Ramsey and Kenneth Beesley

12. Health Security for Rural Poor: Study of Community-Based Health Insurance System in India 177
Sudha Menon

13. Community-Based Hospital: An Alternative Healthcare Arrangement for the Rural Poor in West Bengal 195
Srabanti Chakravarti and Kaushik Chakraborty

14. The Farmer Field School: A Method for Enhancing the Role of Rural Communities in Malaria Control? 213
Henk van den Berg and Bart GJ Knols

• *Index* 225

Overview

There are many ways in which we can define the term 'rural' such as by density of populations, by geographic location and so on. With a plethora of choices in its definition, different parties may disagree with one another quite often on which definition to apply. In the province of healthcare, rural areas can be construed as conspicuous by their suffering from under-serviced delivery owing to a lack of or mal-distribution of resources in terms of money as well as labor. Another characteristic feature of rural health can be noted in the absence of specialty services. Healthcare specialists may not have enough 'critical mass' of patients so as to allow them serve an area with low population in rural areas. There can be demanding hardship on patients in some illnesses that require treatment involving regular long distance travel.

The image of any rural area is that fashioned largely by the city dwellers, who view the countryside as the frequent welcome antithesis of urbanity. Though in some parts of the world, rural life is not the predominant one any more, its influence is visible in suburban yards, city parks and the urban resident's recreational activities. Rural values supposedly provide stability against a rapidly changing modern life. For as long as they lived in cities, people have viewed rural lands normally as their opposites that are primitive yet also unspoiled. In ancient Rome, the distinction cut in two directions that praised urban refinement and yet admitting the fact that rural life was devoid of crime and disease, both too common in cities[1].

All over the world, rural communities often show attributes similar to their neighbors and are consistently found to face an array of problems linked to the international phenomenon of rural decline and urban drift. For instance, it is widely noted that rural populations have poor health status and aging populations. In some parts of the world, multiple state and national policies and programs have been there to redress such a situation. As evidences suggest, the obstacles that healthcare providers and patients face in rural areas are different from those in urban areas a great deal. Rural people often face a unique set of factors creating disparities in healthcare that are absent in urban areas. Economic factors, socio-cultural differences, educational inadequacies, and living in isolated and remote areas often conspire to impede rural people in leading a normal, healthy life. Experts often urge that rural women should especially be given the responsibility of development programs that relate to drinking water, nutrition and primary education to ensure success in any rural health intervention. Traditional healing practices make an integral as well as important component of rural healthcare by virtue of their being the immediate fall back option in most rural settings. Therefore, they need adequate attention especially in the case of any fresh rural health initiative. Modern technologies such as telemedicine have been showing prospects of taking global rural health strides forward.

Lack of availability of health professionals or inadequacy of the same is a major impeding factor concerning rural health. While documenting on 'Prevention of Mother-to-Child Transmission of HIV (PMTCT)', in rural Zimbabwe, Perez *et al.,* (2008) recently pointed out that although the long-term provision concerning Ante-Natal Care (ANC) should be

---

1 Howarth W, The Value of Rural Life in American Culture, *Rural Development Perspectives,* vol. 12, no. 1, accessed on December 22, 2008 from *http://www.ers.usda.gov/publications/rdp/rdp1096/rdp1096b.pdf*

in skilled attendants' hands, encouraging the participation of Trained Birth Attendants (TBAs) in public health programs could help enhance the coverage of mother-child healthcare. They argue that such approach has ample potential to prevent missing of opportunities especially in the case of a significant number of pregnant women in rural areas resorting to home deliveries. Besides, implementation of complex treatment regimens requires on-site availability of drugs as well as the assessing ability of the attendants[2].

Healthcare administrators, researchers and thinkers always get tempted to experiment with innovative approaches to apply in rural areas that can not only counter the challenges of resource scarcity (scarcity of skilled human resources in particular), but also optimize the results in remote settings. Community health workers play an important role in rural healthcare, especially in the decentralized programmatic implications. In developing countries, a major challenge is to make the use of human resources in rural areas including TBAs over and above the challenge to plan as well as implement a definite strategy for public health based on essential care that the skilled attendants provide. Identification of the roles that community workers like TBAs perform can help in facilitating the strategies for improving mother-and-child health when other strategies such as upgradation of existing lower-level facilities, improvement and building of referral systems, supervision and training are considered. Here, it is also necessary to adopt those health policies that legitimize the practice of TBAs instead of coercing and integrating such practices into specific health programs[3].

With innovations, there is an ever-increasing number of possible ways to improve healthcare services in rural areas. Though there is a profusion of literature on making healthcare programs integrated, interdisciplinary

---

2 World Health Organization. 2006. Antiretroviral drugs for treating pregnant women and preventing HIV infection in infants in resource-limited settings. Towards universal access. Recommendations for a public health approach. WHO. Geneva: accessed on February 12, 2007 from *http://www.who.int/hiv/pub/guidelines/pmtctguidelines3.pdf*

3 Perez F, K D Aung, T Ndoro, B Engelsmannand F Dabis, 2008. Participation of traditional birth attendants in prevention of mother-to-child transmission of HIV services in two rural districts in Zimbabwe: a feasibility study, *BMC Public Health*, 8:401, accessed on December 22, 2008 from *http://www.biomedcentral.com/content/pdf/1471-2458-8-401.pdf*

and managed in order to reduce fragmentation and improve continuity and coordination of care, only a small portion of it relates to rural issues. Another challenge is to develop an evidence-based understanding of rural healthcare. An assessment of evidences suggest that the development of new forms of interaction like interdisciplinary and team-based work with flexibility of roles and responsibilities, delegation of tasks and cultural adjustments is particularly relevant in rural areas. Besides, programs like integrated and managed care pathways, outreach programs, shared care and telemedicine are relevant initiatives. Such initiatives may have an association with greater equity in access to care, and more coherent services with greater continuity. A well-functioning system of primary healthcare mostly forms the basis of such endeavors.

Another feature of many rural settings is that the main killer diseases, especially of children that manifest as "acute febrile illness", yet are curable if managed timely and adequately. While introducing a research outcome in the context of rural Uganda, Hildenwall (2008) pointed out that the steps essential to avoid a fatal consequence of such illnesses are: recognition of illness, decision to seek care, reaching an appropriate source by the caretakers and finally receive appropriate treatment. Whenever there is a fatal consequence, some of these steps or all fail and the extent of causation of these outcomes owing to native perception of disease, inappropriate care-seeking or resource inadequacy in the health system or in the family remains to be elucidated. Hildenwall's study explored care-seeking experiences for childhood febrile illness to elucidate the barriers to adequate care that are most influential. Their final identification includes: 1) "Illness interpretation barriers" that involve children who received either delayed or inappropriate care owing to the way caretakers labeled the illness 2) "Barriers to seeking care" with domestic financial constraints and gender roles impeding adequate care 3) "Barriers to receiving adequate treatment" that reveal discontent with providers and likely insufficiencies in quality of care. At the individual as well as health system levels, resource constraints are identified as the causal theme for adequate management. Though the management of severe childhood illness in rural setting has a number of shortcomings, with the children normally seen by an allopathic healthcare provider during the final stage of their illness, improvements of basic healthcare are likely to contribute substantially to reduction of fatal outcomes. Therefore, training support and supply of equipment should be there for the healthcare providers at all levels so that basic healthcare can be enabled for children who suffer from common illnesses[4].

Another major challenge in rural healthcare is the retention of community doctors in remote areas. Like the other professions, the unmatched amenities in urban areas always allure the health professionals in the rural areas to opt for an irreversible migration into the former. This has led to the problem of staffing of rural and remote health centers all over the world more than ever, and this particularly affects sub-Saharan African countries in the present-day context[5].

According to a recent analysis by Dormael *et al.,* (2008), while there has been an increasing attraction of health professionals (doctors) to rural settings in countries like Mali, there is a grave concern for their retention. In 2003, an orientation course was set up for the country's young practicing rural doctors by a professional association in collaboration with a Non-Governmental Organization (NGO) with the underlying assumption that training programs that are rurally relevant would strengthen doctors' competences as well as self-confidence, improve their job satisfaction, and as a result contribute to their retention. While the acceptance of incentive packages condition to work in remote rural areas has been found, the doctors' self-esteem and confidence affect decisions largely to remain in such posts. Appropriate training is found to hopefully contribute to retention by improvement of skills, enhancing self-confidence and changing attitudes. However, other support mechanisms are also required to help practitioners so that they cope with social as well as professional isolation in an effective way[6].

---

4 Hildenwall H, G Thomson, J Kaija, G Pariyo and S Peterson, 2008. "I never had the money for blood testing" – Caretakers' experiences of care-seeking for fatal childhood fevers in rural Uganda – a mixed methods study, *BMC International Health and Human Rights*, 8:12, accessed on December 22, 2008 from *http://www.biomedcentral.com/content/pdf/1472-698X-8-12.pdf*

5 Lehmann, U, M Dieleman M and T Martineau, 2008. Staffing remote rural areas in middle-and low-income countries: a literature review of attraction and retention. *BMC Health Services Research,* 8: 19.

6 Dormael M V, S Dugas, Y Kone, S Coulibaly, M Sy, B Marchal, D Desplats, 2008. Appropriate training and retention of community doctors in rural areas: a case study from Mali, *Human Resources for Health,* 6:25.

The present book is expected to provide a lucid understanding about the issues mentioned and other issues of rural health. It intends to identify the issues and initiatives that portray how government policies, health and community services, population characteristics, local peculiarities and others concerned play their respective roles in addressing the rural health issues and redressing the same as per expediency.

The book is structured into the following two sections:

Section I: **Dimensions**

Section II: **Practices**

As the section titles suggest, the first one deals essentially with conceptual and generic issues accommodating the rationale behind an exclusive consideration for rural health, current trends in rural health that encompass traditional ones like ethnomedicine as well as modern technologies like e-Healthcare and telemedicine. The second section deals with the specific examples of practices all over the world.

The first article titled "**Rural Health: Current Dimensions**" by *Azmal Hussain* discusses the provinces of rural healthcare in the present-day context, including traditional as well as modern practices. Traditional practices include among others "knowledge and beliefs" incorporating plant, animal and/or mineral-based medicines, spiritual therapies, manual techniques and exercises applied singularly or in combination to maintain well-being, as well as to treat, diagnose or prevent illness. Traditional practices have been the sole healthcare means in the case of large part of the world, especially where mainstream healthcare services including western medicine are not available. One sub-section of the article is focused on telehealth, which is introduced like other Information and Communication Technologies (ICTs) to support the delivery of healthcare services. It is presently being considered as a viable means to answer many imperatives that currently challenge healthcare systems. Traditional healing practices make an integral as well as important component of rural healthcare by virtue of their being the immediate fall back option in most rural settings. Therefore, they need adequate attention especially in the case of any fresh rural health initiative. Likewise, modern technologies such as telemedicine have been showing prospects of taking global rural health strides forward.

The next article "**Rural Health Insurance: A Hope for the Poor**" by *Azmal Hussain,* focuses on health insurance as a vehicle for healthcare transformation in rural areas. The importance of healthcare in rural areas and the benefits of health insurance at various stages of life demand special attention, considering the low levels of literacy and inefficiency. The cost of medical care for those people who do not have insurance coverage may extend ranging from a small financial cost to a catastrophic expenditure. Rural health insurance (RHI) has been an effective means of saving rural poor from having to make catastrophic payments. RHI can contribute in improving rural livelihood in many other ways. To demonstrate its efficacy, examples from a number of success stories have been presented.

The third article titled "**Chronic Disease Management Systems (Registries) in Rural Health Care**" by *Anne Skinner, Roslyn Fraser-Maginn* and *Keith J Mueller* is about Chronic Disease Management Systems (CDMS), a tool that helps providers efficiently collect and analyze patient information to promote quality care for rural population. A CDMS is a patient-centered electronic database tool that helps providers diagnose, treat and manage chronic diseases. Citing evidences from the US, the authors point out that CDMS can be made available to rural clinics and implemented as well as maintained by clinic staff with minimal technological expenditures. Healthcare providers can use CDMS to capture and track scientific processes and outcome indicators related to the care of a patient diagnosed with a chronic disease. Finally, for an effective and sustainable change, implementation of CDMS should be accompanied by change in clinical processes, incorporation of interdisciplinary service and patients' participation.

The fourth article titled "**A Web-Based Graphical User Interface for Evidence-Based Decision-Making for Health Care Allocations in Rural Areas**" by *Nadine Schuurman, Margo Leight* and *Myriam Berube* talks about the policy-makers who are increasingly recognizing the importance of evidence-based decision-making – based on integrating results from the best available systematic research with seasoned professional judgment and expertise. Evidence-Based Decision-Making (EBDM) requires a commitment of resources to support the identification of pertinent questions and the research initiatives most appropriate to answer them. This article deals with a Web-based Graphical User Interface (GUI) to assist health policy makers and administrators to make well-informed decisions about the location and allocation of time-sensitive service capacities in rural areas. This tool integrates datasets for existing hospitals and services, regional populations and road networks to allow users to ascertain the percentage of population in any given service catchment who are served by a specific health service, or baskets of linked services. The GUI allows policy-makers to map trauma and obstetric services against rural populations within pre-specified travel distances, illustrating service capacity by region. The authors conclude that the interfaces can be used by health policy-makers and administrators with little or no formal GIS training to visualize multiple health resource allocation scenarios.

The succeeding article titled "**Bridging Rural Health Research and Policy: Dissemination Strategies**" by *Keith J Mueller, Timothy D McBride, Andrew F Coburn, Rebecca T Slifkin, Mary K Wakefield* and *A Clinton MacKinney* describes five strategies that are considered as critical to effective dissemination and expanded use of rural health services research. These include the need for researchers and funders to do the following: engage end users when framing research; tailor the design of products to meet the diverse needs of the end users interested in rural health research; make research products easily accessible to end users; expand contact and working relationships with end users and invest in developing greater capacity for effective dissemination. Over and above, the article discusses the infrastructure needed to enhance research dissemination. Researchers earn the trust of policy makers when they: present accurate and evidence-based information; acknowledge data or information limitations; provide an objective and nonpartisan viewpoint; work diligently to be recognized experts in their field; respond to user requests in a timely fashion and provide policy-relevant information specific to user needs. Users' need for immediate, relevant and quality research when the policy is being developed and not after the fact requires that researchers develop an ability to adapt to the needs of users if they want their research to be valued and used.

The sixth article titled "**National Centre of Rural Medicine in Norway: A Bridge from Rural Practice to the Academy**" by *IJ Aaraas* and *E Swensen* is the first in section II, and discusses the aims and achievements of National Center for Rural Medicine (NCRM) in Norway. The NCRM was dedicated to examining both common and diverse expressions and values of rural practice, and to use this insight and knowledge to revitalize and strengthen the healthcare provided to rural population. Among the three major activities and achievements of NCRM, the first is in the form of published descriptions and distinctions of rural medicine to encourage national collegial discussion about the concept and nature of rural medicine. The second is a professional development and research program constituting a varied portfolio of themes. The third major achievement is an innovation of networking and meeting places for rural practitioners aimed at enhancing opportunities to share experiences, build theory and discuss professional development issues.

The subsequent article titled "**Quality through Collaboration: The Future of Rural & Frontier Emergency Medical Services in the US Health System**" is sourced from the US Department of Health and Human Services and Administration Office of Rural Health Policy (HRSA). It initially discusses how improving the quality of healthcare services has become a key focus of the healthcare industry, State and Federal government payers, commercial insurers, employers, and increasingly, patients and the general public in the context of the US. Subsequently, five strategies to address the quality challenges in rural communities are discussed. The first strategy is to adopt an integrated, priority approach to address both personal and population health needs at the community level. The second strategy is to establish a stronger quality improvement support structure for rural health systems and professionals for acquiring knowledge and tools to improve quality. The next is to enhance the human resource capacity of rural communities, including education, training and deployment of health care professionals, and the preparedness of rural residents to engage actively in improving their health and health care. The fourth strategy is to monitor rural health care systems to ensure that they are financially stable and provide assistance in securing the necessary capital for system redesign. The last strategy is to invest in building Information and Communication Technology (ICT) infrastructure, which has enormous potential to enhance health and health care over the coming decade.

The following article titled "**Rural Health Insurance – Rising to the Challenge**" is sourced from the *World Bank*. It focuses on the challenges of rural health insurance in China and documents some responses at the government level. Rising to the challenge, China's Government recently developed plans for a New Cooperative Medical Scheme (NCMS). The new county level scheme has also been initiated against the backdrop of an almost total collapse of the old village-level rural Cooperative Medical Scheme (CMS). Both the programs face challenges relating to breadth and depth of coverage, cost control, quality assurance and so on. China's central government has also seen increases in its tax revenues, and is committed to spending some of them on rural health, in general, and on the NCMS, in particular.

The ninth article titled "**Telemedicine in Rural India**" by *Sanjit Bagchi* discusses the prospects and challenges of telemedicine in rural India, with special focus on Indian Space Research Organization's (ISRO) telemedicine initiative. The efficacy of telemedicine has already been shown through the network established by ISRO, which has connected 22 super-specialty hospitals with 78 rural and remote hospitals across the country through its geo-stationary satellites. The network initiated by ISRO has reportedly enabled thousands of patients in remote places like Jammu and Kashmir, Andaman and Nicobar Islands, the Lakshadweep Islands, and tribal areas of the central and northeastern regions of India to gain access to consultations with experts in super-specialty medical institutions. The author cautions that telemedicine initiative in rural India has not been free of challenges that are posed to any new technology due to people's unfamiliarity. For instance, though the systems are user-friendly, there are people who are affected by the fear of the unknown in handling computers and other equipment. However, such difficulties of technophobia can be surmounted, and the country's telemedicine initiative has the potential to provide specialized health care to millions of poor Indians.

The subject matter of the tenth article titled "**Pre-Triage Procedures in Mobile Rural Health Clinics in Ethiopia**" by *PC Stillman* and *PC Strong* is on a series of mobile health clinics sponsored by an indigenous relief organization in rural Ethiopia. In coordinating with local health authorities, the purpose of these clinics was to provide acute care medical treatment and public health teaching. An important step in the intervention was a 'pre-triage' process that had evolved over a series of previous rural mobile clinic trips, and then involving lead physicians and nurse-translators moving through the crowd selecting prospective patients. Subsequently, a process developed that *inter alia* involved modification of the pre-triage process by involving more people in patient selection. In subsequent clinics, this new process was well accepted and contributed to increased efficiency and an overall improved community outreach. An important learning from the intervention is that setting expectations regarding the purpose of the mobile clinic and the scope of the problems that could be treated are essential, which are best done at the outset of the clinic in coordination with local health authorities.

The succeeding article titled "**Rural Community Well-Being: The Perspectives of Health Care Managers in Southwestern Manitoba, Canada**" by *Doug Ramsey* and *Kenneth Beesley* discusses the perspectives of rural healthcare managers regarding rural community well-being. Healthcare issues in rural areas are many and varied in the western world including an aging population and rural depopulation. Many parts of rural Canada are facing declining populations, making the case for designating healthcare resources more difficult. The authors provide a conceptual framework in the context of rural community well-being and apply the same within a Canadian Regional Health Authority. The framework proves useful in identifying determinants of health as well as assessing the role of social capacity in fostering rural community well-being.

Section I

Dimensions

Like many other livelihood challenges, rural people face a range of health problems that are conspicuously different from those faced in urban areas. The main challenge facing the rural and remote communities is arguably the accessibility to vital health services. Particularly in the developing world, rural communities are mostly characterized by prevailing issues like low literacy level, low health level, resource constraints and professional isolation. Rural populations normally witness higher rates of illness coupled with less access to healthcare resources. At that health insurance coverage is much lower in rural areas than urban areas. These factors and many more necessitate identification and addressing of the healthcare needs of rural communities so that the findings can be contextualized in wider rural health environment. This article discusses the current dimensions of rural health encompassing the various provinces of rural healthcare in the present-day context, including traditional as well as modern practices. The major health challenges facing the rural world are also discussed in possible details.

2. Rural Health: Some Major Issues

2.1 Rising Healthcare Costs: Implications for Rural Healthcare

Recently, rural healthcare expenditures have been rising thereby causing a burden for rural communities as well as the others concerned. Several factors can be held responsible for rising healthcare expenditures, such as changes in the healthcare needs of the population, changing socioeconomic status, changes in provider price, and technological changes to top it all. Rural areas disproportionately get affected by these factors whereupon strategies to contain surge in healthcare expenditure may need to be different in rural settings and may be done best on a local basis. Rising healthcare costs are a grave concern to rural people, rural employers, taxpayers, legislators and so on[1].

Rural decision-makers need to consider the factors contributing mostly to rising healthcare spending. They should also consider whether and how such factors are poised to change in time to come. Some rural-specific considerations

---

1 Strunk B C & P B Ginsburg, 2004. *Tracking healthcare costs: Spending growth slowdown stalls in first half of 2004* (Issue Brief 91). Washington, DC: Center for Studying Health System Change.

pertinent to these factors may include the following *inter alia*[2]: change in healthcare needs of the rural population; economic changes concerning income and wages; changes in provider price; and technological change.

2.2 Rural Health Insurance: Feasibility Challenges

Inadequate health insurance almost goes synonymously with poor rural communities. This compounds the already deplorable health situation in many rural areas. The brunt of taxation that rural families have to bear often turns catastrophic. In this context, an example from rural Cambodia is seemingly pertinent. Among the Southeast Asian countries, Cambodia happens to be the worst sufferer of infant, childhood and maternal mortality, and the country's health problem gets compounded by dengue fever, which causes substantial out-of-pocket expenses besides creating substantial socio-economic burden for families. There is evidence suggesting that perceptions of mothers regarding the healthcare cost and financial constraints result in considerable delays in seeking healthcare[3]. Drawing on in-depth interviews with mothers of children who were infected with dengue in the country's eastern part, Khun and Manderson illustrated the deep economic consequences for households in case of a child's illness. The introduction of user fees in the country's public health facilities in 1997 was intended to enhance service quality through injection of funds into the existing health system. As health insurance was not adequate, a scheme of social safety net was introduced so that all people could attend the health facilities. However, continuing high hospitalization rates and mortality from dengue among infants and children portrayed the difficulties that women faced in finding enough cash in cases of emergency, resulting in delays both in diagnosis and treatment. The direct costs for healthcare and medical services, coupled with added indirect costs caused poor women to deter from providing healthcare to their ailing children. Those who eventually sought healthcare had to incur health spending often through loans and out-of-pocket payments, or sold property, essential goods or labor to meet the expenses that were catastrophic at times, exacerbating the

---

2 McBride T D, 2005. Why are Healthcare Expenditures Increasing and is there a Rural Differential? *Rural Policy Brief,* 10 (7): RUPRI Center for Rural Health Policy Analysis.

3 Khun S & L Manderson, 2007. Health seeking and access to care for children with suspected dengue in Cambodia: An ethnographic study., *BMC Public Health,* 7: 262.

2.5 Health Surveillance for Rural Areas

Population-based sample surveys along with sentinel surveillance methods commonly act as substitutes for health and demographic studies on intervention and monitoring in resource-poor rural settings. However, such methods often face criticisms worldwide for being worthwhile only in case of any possibility of extrapolation of the results to the surrounding 100-fold population. Still, evidence from diverse rural settings suggests that sample surveys can provide useful insights in demographic as well as health profiles of native rural populations, and to ensure cost-effectiveness such surveys should be representative enough so as to be generalized to the surrounding population. Strategies of sampling thus need adequate consideration, but it is a big challenge to ascertain that a particular sampling method best represents various parameters under measurement and their distribution in the sampling unit. Therefore, it is likely that compromises may need to be made while choosing a sampling strategy. It is not always true that simple approaches to sampling are always less appropriate compared to more complex ones. In fact the simpler ones, needing less specialist expertise, are able to provide much useful information relevant to local public health planning, their implementation, monitoring and evaluation[9]. Besides, for improving rural peoples' health status, community-based action research in combination with critical ethnography is viewed as a constructive approach[10].

3. Traditional Practices in Rural Healthcare

Traditional healing practices make an integral as well as important component of rural healthcare by virtue of their being the immediate fall back option in most rural settings. These practices include among others traditional knowledge and beliefs incorporating living objects like plants and animals and/or inanimate ones including spiritual therapies, mineral based medicines, and manual techniques as well as exercises that are applied either in combination or singularly to maintain well-being, besides treating, diagnosing or preventing illness. Traditional practices

---

9 Fottrell E and P Byass, 2008. Population survey sampling methods in a rural African setting: measuring mortality, *Population Health Metrics*, 6:2, accessed on November 21, 2008 from *http://www.pophealthmetrics.com/content/6/1/2*

10 Averill J B, 2006. Getting Started: Initiating Critical Ethnography and Community-based Action Research in a Program of Rural Health Studies, *International Journal of Qualitative Methods* 5 (2).

have been the sole healthcare means in case of large part of the world, especially where the mainstream healthcare services including Western medicine are not available.

Despite many strides made by modern systems of medicine, traditional or local medicine remains an important means of medical care even today in many developing countries. This is despite the lack of official recognition from the government level healthcare programs in these countries. In some areas, both in rural and urban settings this persists along with allopathic health services[11,12]. Due to this and several other factors, traditional healing practices have gained so much of contemporary relevance especially in rural areas[13]. Historically, traditional healing practices and rural health have been going on hand-in-hand. There is a plethora of research findings delineating traditional medicinal practices prevailing in rural and remote areas all over the world. Traditional herbal therapies as well as traditional complimentary and alternative medicines are commonly used in African countries by public health facilities' HIV treatment naïve outpatients. As concluded by a recent study by Peltzer *et al.,* in South Africa, healthcare providers should screen patients on use of traditional complimentary and alternative medicines when initiating antiretroviral therapy and during follow-up as well as monitoring, keeping in view that these patients might not disclose other therapies fully. Co-location of various services, including voluntary associations that offer spiritual and/or holistic healthcare advice, may help in addressing patients' needs where healthcare providers lack the knowledge or time to address these issues effectively[14].

The importance of traditional healing practices is manifold. Particularly, in remote rural areas of Africa, Latin America and Asia, more so among tribal

---

11 Bhasin, V. 2007. "Medical Anthropology: A Review". *Studies on Ethnomedicine.* 1 (1): 1-20.

12 Kleinman, A. 1980. Patients and Healers in the Context of Culture: An Exploration of the Borderland between Anthropology, Medicine and Psychiatry. Berkeley: University California Press.

13 Hussain, A 2008. Conceptualizing ethnomedicine: Current dimensions, In A Hussain (ed), *Ethnomedicine: Global Perspectives,* Icfai University Press, Hyderabad.

14 Peltzer K, N Friend-du Preez, S Ramlagan, H Fomundam and J Anderson, 2008. Use of Traditional Complementary and Alternative Medicine (TCAM) by HIV patients prior to initiating ART in KwaZulu-Natal, South Africa, *Journal of the International AIDS Society,* 11(Suppl 1):P73 accessed on November 22, 2008 from *http://www.jiasociety.org/content/11/S1/P73*

Mouka *et al.* (2008) concluded that the fundamental principles in managing a psychiatric case should be that the patient gets what s/he needs, when s/he needs it and where is the best possibility of getting it. Evidence also suggests increased needs of community-based rural mental health services and that a community-centric program based on mobile rural psychiatric units offers quite satisfactory results towards this end[24].

It is generally believed that Information and Communication Technology (ICT) has a tendency to provide manifold solutions for health problems through e-Healthcare technologies. The nature of information can be improved to a great deal by healthcare professionals through the use of ICT in day-to-day patient care[25]. Emerging fields like e-Healthcare is considered as an outcome of the overwhelming acceptance gained by ICT in the modern province of healthcare. However, in many developing countries, ICT projects are allegedly associated with failure, owing mainly to contextual, operational and strategy constraints. A substantial ICT improvement in the field of healthcare is currently represented by e-Healthcare, and its failure as such can lead to huge losses in effort, money and time[26].

Recently, a model called "shared resources solution" has come into surface, which uses emerging "utility grid technology" that acts as an enabler for the provisioning of ubiquitous e-Healthcare service. As the supporters claim, the approach has enormous potential to brink a number of positive changes in rural healthcare such as: to improve time to treatment; to promote evidence-based management; to provide support for proactive care and point-of-care treatment; to empower consumers by ensuring accessibility of healthcare services through mobile devices; and to facilitate provider-consumer interaction. However, cooperation and adequate exchange of information among the disparate as well as dispersed healthcare organizations are necessary for the success of shared care.

24 Mouka V, V Peritogiannis, M Lekka, M Nepheli, Mavreas Venetsanos and T Hyphantis, 2008. The development of a mobile psychiatric unit in a rural area of Greece: preliminary results, *Annals of General Psychiatry* , 7(Suppl 1), accessed on November 21, 2008 from *http://www.annals-general-psychiatry.com/content/7/S1/S280*

25 Katehakis D G, M Tsiknakis and S C Orphanoudakis, 2002. A healthcare information infrastructure to support integrated services over regional health telematics network. *Health IT Advisory Report,* 4 (1): 15-18.

26 Van B J H & M A Musen (ed.), 1997. *Handbook of Medical Informatics.* A W Houten. Springer Velag.

Economic incentives for the participants are also required for the sustainability of this cooperation and information exchange[27].

Like e-Healthcare, telemedicine is another popular term in the modern province of rural healthcare. To put in simple words, telemedicine is "the use of electronic information and communications technologies to provide and support healthcare when distance separates the participants"[28]. It has impacted the delivery of rural healthcare services a great deal in recent times. In the US, federal as well as state governments have invested ample support amounts in the form of incentives, infrastructure and equipment for consumers as well as providers so that the use of telecommunications can be expanded in medical care in the right earnest. Experts urge that if telemedicine can establish itself as a useful tool to improve the possibility of rural hospitals' survival, then it can be a technology in the greater interest of rural development. Supporters also argue that telemedicine has enormous potential to address several problems simultaneously characterizing rural healthcare that includes quality assurance access to care and cost containment. Access can be improved amply by establishing linkage between providers in remote areas and specialists in metropolitan centers. Over and above adding effect of retention status among healthcare professionals in remote areas, telemedicine enables a wider service outreach in the local community. It can also promote cost containment by substituting lower-cost rural healthcare providers and facilities[29]. However, all such prospects are subject to thorough evaluation.

5. Conclusion

Rural people face a number of health challenges, which are conspicuously different from what urban people face concerning the nature as well as extent. This makes rural health as a discrete discipline to be dealt with differently from urban health. Health insurance, hospitals with adequate infrastructure, human resources for

---

27 Buyya R and S Venugopal, 2004. *The Gridbus Toolkit for Service Oriented Grid and Utility Computing: An Overview and Status Report* [presented at the first IEEE International Workshop on Grid Economics and Business Models, GECON].

28 Capalbo S N & Heggem C N, 1999. Evaluating Telemedicine Technologies in Rural Settings, Policy Issues Paper No. 10, USDA National Agricultural Library, Community Development resources, accessed on Novemebr 24 from *http://www2.montana.edu/jantle/trc/pdf/policypapers/pp10.pdf*

29 *Ibid.*

health, and many other essential healthcare elements are relatively scarce in case of rural areas, whereupon people's fate in rural areas is reasonably more precarious. In remote rural areas of the world, cases of varied ailments are presented to traditional healers, whereupon traditional healing practices become a very pertinent healthcare issue amidst the inadequacy or absence of conventional healthcare services in those areas. While traditional practices have been the sole healthcare means in case of large part of the rural world, modern healing practices should also go hand-in-hand with the traditional ones to take rural health steps forward.

Rural decision-makers need to consider the factors that contribute mostly to rising healthcare spending as well as the possibilities of whether and how such factors are poised to change in time to come. Change in healthcare needs of the rural population, economic changes concerning income and wages, changes in provider price, and technological change can be some of these options. Expanding health insurance coverage in rural areas would enormously benefit the low-income rural residents, over and above reinforcing the overall system of rural health by increasing revenues of healthcare provider thereby helping other rural folk. Understanding health insurance patterns among remote rural communities is also important as it can help immensely while designing rural insurance reform strategies in the health sector.

For some common vaccine-preventable diseases, efforts to increase immunization coverage in rural areas should be given adequate consideration to the factors contributing to the incomplete immunization status of children. Missed vaccination opportunities as well as incorrect vaccination also need to be avoided in the right earnest so that vaccine coverage can be increased for those reaching the health facility. Such steps are especially relevant in countries where health services lack 100 percent of coverage.

As far as the use of traditional complimentary and alternative medicines is concerned, healthcare providers should make it a point to screen patients when initiating any therapy and during follow-up as well as monitoring, keeping in view that these patients might not disclose other therapies fully. Co-location of various services may as well help in addressing patients' needs if healthcare providers lack the knowledge or time to do so. Lastly, there is also increased need for community-based rural mental health services and a community-centric program based on mobile rural psychiatric units that may offer good results.

(Azmal Hussain, Consulting Editor, Icfai Research Centre, Kolkata. He can be reached at azmalhussain@icfai.org).

2

Rural Health Insurance
A Hope for the Poor

Azmal Hussain

This article is focused on health insurance as a vehicle for healthcare transformation in rural areas. The importance of healthcare in rural areas and the benefits of health insurance at various stages of life demand special attention, considering the low levels of literacy, and inefficiency. The cost of medical care for those people who do not have insurance coverage may extend ranging from a small financial cost to a severe one. Rural Health Insurance (RHI) has been an effective means of saving rural poor from having to make catastrophic payments. RHI can contribute in improving rural livelihood in many other ways. To demonstrate its efficacy, examples from a number of success stories have been presented.

1. Background

In the developing and transition countries, healthcare policy as well as healthcare services are grave concerns especially in rural areas. For many rural communities, the viability may depend a great deal on the range and quality of available healthcare services.[1] One of the gravest public health issues in the developing and underdeveloped areas is lack of health insurance, more so in case of rural areas. Expanding health insurance coverage in rural areas would not only benefit the low-income residents, but also would reinforce the overall system of rural health by increasing revenues of healthcare provider thereby helping other rural folk. Research indicates that people in rural areas are less likely to be insured compared to their urban counterparts. Understanding health insurance patterns among rural communities can be of help while designing insurance reform strategies in the health sector that can build on existing rural health service coverage. Evidences also suggest that rural people, particularly those who live in remotest places, are at the greatest risk of being uninsured. Such likelihood imposes a much greater financial vulnerability of rural communities to medical costs than any other population[2]. With this background, the article attempts to discuss health insurance as a vehicle for healthcare transformation in rural areas.

2. Trends in Rural Health Insurance: A Generic View

Recent paper headlines across the world often talk about the ever-increasing healthcare costs and the attendant relevance of health insurance. Hundreds of millions of people cannot afford health insurance in such a situation, and the number of such unfortunates is still growing. The problem is more acute in rural areas as rural people by and large tend to be poorer and rural households are more prone to have incomes lying below the general poverty level. Furthermore, the healthcare infrastructure is by and large more fragile and resources are more scarce in rural settings than the urban ones. The income disparity is even more pronounced for rural minorities. Therefore, while seeking solutions to rural people's health insurance access, some unique rural characteristics as well as circumstances must be given due consideration so that unintended consequences may be avoided in the right earnest. Any policy remedy to the absence or dearth of health insurance in rural areas should also be sensitive to such characteristics of rural life[3].

1 United States Department of Agriculture (USDA), 2007. Rural Healthcare and Health Insurance (Farm Bill Forum Comment Summary and Background) [accessed on October 7, 2008 from *http://www.usda.gov/documents/RURAL_HEALTH_CARE_AND_HEALTH_ INSURANCE.pdf*].

2 Maine Rural Health Research Center, 2007. Rural Families More Likely to be Uninsured and have Different Sources of Coverage, Research & Policy Brief, Muskie School of Public Service [accessed on October 7, 2008 from *http://muskie.usm.maine.edu/Publications/rural/pb34.pdf*].

3 Colorado Rural Health Council. Issue Paper: Health Insurance Access in Rural Colorado January 2003, accessed on November 13, 2008 from *http://www.coruralhealth.org/crhc/resources/publications/issuepapers/insurance_access12.06.pdf*

Over the last decade, several studies have documented rural residents' lower rates of coverage of health insurance than their urban counterparts[4,5,6]. Such difference is attributed largely to the fact that people in rural areas have very limited access to coverage based on private employers owing to their tendency to work for smaller firms thereby earning lower wages than their urban counterparts[7]. In many an instance, rural residents work in sectors like agriculture, fishing, forestry, or allied ones that are not quite likely to offer any health insurance sponsored by private employers. Again, sometimes owing to sub-optimal productivity many rural residents may opt for multiple seasonal or part-time jobs, which can further lower the job-related coverage[8]. On top of these, in rural areas, average incomes are usually lower when compared to urban ones that further tend to depress insurance coverage. Among low income rural families, establishing or enhancing insurance coverage can raise revenues for rural health facilities, practitioners and other healthcare providers. The burden owing to uncompensated care like treating uninsured individuals can be reduced by doing this. This can also facilitate a situation where providers can continue to render services to other patients including those with private insurance[9].

Thus, for many people in developing countries "health insurance" is quite an unknown word. The general assumption is that, barring the upper classes, people in the developing world can hardly afford social protection of such type. This is a pity as poor people also demand for protection against various financial consequences of illnesses. It is true for most rural poor in developing countries that illness represents a permanent threat even today to their capacity to earn income. Over and above the direct treatment and medicine costs, indirect costs

4 Ziller, E, A Coburn, S Loux, C Hoffman, & T McBride, 2003. *Health Insurance Coverage in Rural America: A Chartbook.* Washington, D.C.: Kaiser Family Foundation, Kaiser Commission on Medicaid and the Uninsured.

5 Larson, S.L. & S C Hill, 2005. Rural-urban differences in employment-related health insurance. *Journal of Rural Health, Winter, 21* (1): 21-30.

6 Pol, L. (2000). "Health insurance in Rural America." Rural Policy Brief 5(11). RUPRI Center for Rural Health Policy Analysis.

7 Coburn, AF, E H Kilbreth, S H Long, & M S Marquis, 1998. Urban-rural differences in employer-based health insurance coverage of workers. *Medical Care Research and Review, 55* (4), 484-96).

8 National Rural Health Association, "Access to Healthcare for the Uninsured in Rural and Frontier America," Kansas City, MO, 1999.

9 Centre for Budget and Policy Priorities, 2001. Improving Rural Parents' Health Insurance Coverage: A Fact Sheet, accessed on November 17, 2008 from *http://www.cbpp.org/7-25-01health-fact3.htm*

to the households owing to the ill person's missing labor force along with that of the occupying person causes many a hardship.

Of late, however, in low income countries, health insurance schemes are increasingly being recognized as a tool to finance healthcare provision. Amidst the sky-scraping latent demand from the public for good quality healthcare services and the utter under-utilization of healthcare services in many countries, it is often argued that schemes like social health insurance can improve healthcare access of acceptable quality. While alternative strategies of healthcare financing and cost recovery such as user fees often face severe criticisms, the option of insurance is seemingly a promising alternative owing to its being a possibility to pool transferring of risks and unforeseeable costs of healthcare to fixed premiums. In recent past, mainly the countries of Sub-Saharan Africa along with a number of other countries have largely witnessed the emergence of mutual, community-based non-profit health insurance schemes. An ethic of solidarity, mutual aid and collective mechanism of pooling health risks makes the hallmark of such schemes, which operate in several countries in conjunction with the providers of healthcare especially in native hospitals. Here, it is pertinent to take note of the analyses by the 'Center for Development Research (ZEF-Bonn)' within its research program on rural social security systems that dealt with the challenges as well as prospects of innovative schemes of health insurance. The institute is instrumental in carrying out empirical studies with collaborative support from national research institutes in India, China, Ethiopia, Ghana, Senegal and Tanzania. These projects are aimed at estimating healthcare and health insurance demands, quantifying socioeconomic impacts over and above identifying factors of success as well as failure[10].

As one such study shows, even the rural poor are able to insure themselves against health risks. The study was carried out in the Thiès region of rural Senegal. In the last decade or so, the community based rural health insurance schemes were developed basing on traditional type of mutual assistance. These schemes of mutual health insurance have about 500 members each and are totally routed in the native setting. The crux of idea is that low cost expenditures are borne by the family, whereas the costs are borne by the mutual health insurance in case of

[10] Johannes Jütting, Health insurance for the rural poor ? *http://www.oecd.org/dataoecd/31/38/2510517.pdf*

hospitalization. To do so, a contract has been established by the community-based health insurance schemes with St. Jean de Dieu a church-run hospital in Thiès. The members of the mutual health insurance are granted substantially reduced fees through this contract for specific services and treatments. As suggested by another evaluation in recent past, members of a mutual health insurance have better healthcare access accompanied by benefits in other ways compared to non-members. A member can join the hospital in case of any serious illness more often than non-members and that too by paying half of the amount that any non-member has to pay. The study also documented that joining a mutual health insurance scheme has resulted in a reduction in its members' worries. The members no longer depend on assistance from social networks or money borrowed from the local money-lenders. However, amidst all these encouraging signs, the study has revealed another important fact that due to lack of financial resource required to pay for regular subscription of membership the 'poorest of the poor' hardly participate in the scheme[11].

The most recent opportunity for the rural poor as well as insurance marketers has surfaced in the form of micro-insurance. In countries like India, the majority of the people hail from rural areas with negligible insurance coverage. This lack of insurance coverage is often responsible for catastrophic expenditure, especially health expenditure. Such a situation opens enormous opportunity for marketers of micro-insurance products. If operated sensibly, it can create a win-win solution for the persistent health challenges in rural areas. Micro-insurance is a type of finance designed in such a way that it suits the needs of rural poor who have no access to other conventional forms of insurance. The small premium policies form the hallmark of this type of insurance. Rural people's health needs are different from their counterpart in urban areas and formal insurance products may not be able to fulfill them. In India a service tax of 10.36 percent is imposed for insurance products, but to enhance their penetration in rural areas and to make insurance viable for the villagers, such a high rate of tax should be done away with[12].

---

11 Johannes Jütting, Health insurance for the rural poor ? *http://www.oecd.org/dataoecd/31/38/2510517.pdf*

12 Agarwal A, 2007. Micro-Insurance – Gateway to rural upliftment, accessed on December 23, 2008 from *http://www.labnol.org/india/law/micro-insurance-gateway-to-rural-upliftment/317/*

3. Rural Health Insurance: Some Viability Factors

A multiple of factors need to be at play if any rural health insurance program has to be effective in a given socio-ecological setting. In this context, a number of studies have been conducted in India, Rwanda and Thailand by various research institutes on the effect of risk sharing by the community in healthcare. These studies along with the Senegal case were analyzed by the World Health Organization's (WHO) 'Commission on Macroeconomics and Health' to examine the interrelations among economic growth, investment in health, and poverty reduction[13,14]. Some important findings of the various studies regarding the scheme design may be summarized as under:

3.1 Flexibility in Paying Procedure

The Rwandan experience suggests that the households, who were unable to pay the premium in a single bit, were allowed to do so in easy installments to a tontine prior to joining a pre-payment scheme. Besides, fees were collected by church based groups for the disabled, indigent, orphans and the likes. The Senegal experience also reported contributions from charitable organizations whereupon the people who were otherwise excluded got the chance to take part in the mutual health insurance. Some schemes even start collective activities and earnings accrued there from were used to pay membership fees. In fine, an array of possibilities are there to adapt paying procedures in tune with the local level requirements. The state's roles such as creating options for demand targeted subsidies in this context also merit thorough exploration[15].

3.2 Community Participation and Social Protection

Voluntary not-for-profit organizations acting as intermediaries between the providers' interest and the members' needs and expectations often form community financing schemes. It is of paramount importance to deal with these ambiguities

---

13 Preker A S, G Carrin, D Dror, M Jakab, W Hsiao, & D Arhin-Tenkorang, 2002. Effectiveness of community health financing in meeting the cost of illness, *Bulletin of the World Health Organization*;80:143-150. accessed on November 20, 2008 from *http://whqlibdoc.who.int/bulletin/2002/Vol80-No2/bulletin_2002_80(2)_143-150.pdf*

14 Schieber G. 2005. Sustainable Health Sector Health Sector Financing, (High Level Forum on the Health Level Forum on the Health MDGs MDGs in Asia in Asia-Pacific Pacific), accessed on November 20, 2008 from *http://www.wpro.who.int/NR/rdonlyres/B29DBB95-A09A-4C78-B545-B83D9C8E9662/0/12SustainablehealthsectorfinancingGSchieberWorldBank.pdf*

15 *Ibid.*

whereupon the presence of trained personnel becomes a dire necessity. In this context it needs to be emphasized that to handle the claims the administrative procedure should be simple and transparent in the best possible way. The experience of Bangladesh's Grameen Bank suggest the possibility of better performance by mutual insurance schemes linked to organizations already having experience in the area of social protection and financial services[16].

Community participation does matter, when it comes to cost control and moderation of moral hazard behavior. Empirical evidence suggests that the degree of participation of the community members in the design as well as running of the schemes of community financing can have a wide range of variation and the more the funds are owned as well as managed by the community members themselves the greater is the degree of participation. Conversely, participation is low in case of the schemes run by health facilities. It is quite rational to argue that if the community members are able to identify "their" schemes with themselves by virtue of having the decision-making power and controlling the funds, they will have a normal tendency to lessen unnecessary use of various healthcare services.

3.3 A Viable Healthcare Provider

A health insurance scheme's success or failure largely depends on the presence of a viable healthcare provider such as the hospital offering services to the insured. Mobilization of demand for community financing schemes and their financial schemes are greatly influenced by the providers' decisions. In this respect, the Senegalese experience enlightens: The movement of mutual health organization has been supported right from its inception by St. Jean de Dieu – the church-run hospital. The hospital administration recognized that the poor people, their ultimate target group were not able to pay their fees. It was not possible either for the hospital to consider any exemption of fees. The formation of mutual health organization made it possible to target their clientele directly as well as cost-effectively. Besides, the financial support extended by the hospital to the mutual health

[16] Schieber G. 2005. Sustainable Health Sector Health Sector Financing, (High Level Forum on the Health Level Forum on the Health MDGs MDGs in Asia in Asia-Pacific Pacific), accessed on November 20, 2008 from *http://www.wpro.who.int/NR/rdonlyres/B29DBB95-A09A-4C78-B545-B83D9C8E9662/0/12Sustainablehealthsectorfinancing GSchieberWorldBank.pdf*

organizations accompanied by high quality service delivery is a very important point in mobilizing demand in the long run[17].

3.4 Community and Household Characteristics

If the benefits are to be realized from community financing schemes, a genuine demand for health insurance is of crucial importance. The demand for health insurance from rural households depends on the benefit package, premium, quality of care accessible from the healthcare provider, and cultural and socioeconomic characteristics of the beneficiary communities and households. Pervasive poverty among potential members of a health insurance scheme can be a serious impediment to its implementation. If people struggle for survival day in and day out, they would be willing to pay the essential insurance premiums in advance with the aim of using services at a later time. Even the removal of barriers to access may not stop social exclusion to persist in the population. The same can also be said of exemption mechanisms for the rural poor or sliding premium scales as these are very difficult to implement. Before or after introducing the health insurance, it can be necessary for the development projects to bring about an enhancement of income so that members can get attracted and realize the potential payback of community financing.

The prevailing concepts of risk and illness have their relevance to the households' decision whether or not to purchase health insurance. If illness is perceived by the people as a rather random event that has a chance to hit anyone, then there is more likelihood that the prospective beneficiaries will purchase insurance at their own free will unlike in a condition where people perceive illness as a punishment for misbehavior. Cultural practices in dealing with disease risks can influence insurance demand a great deal. Cultural barriers often act as obstacles to opt for health insurance in remote rural areas as for events like funerals or marriages, people normally put money aside but believe that saving money for meeting eventual healthcare costs means "wishing oneself the disease". If there is a strong solidarity, people do not bother much if the benefits accrued from the premiums they pay would come to themselves or other members in the community. It is a

---

17 Preker *et al., op cit.*

general belief that the degree of solidarity as well as mutual trust is relatively higher in case of close-knit homogeneous communities compared to diverse or scattered populations that comprise people hailing from various religious, cultural and ethnic origin.

Public insurance programs become all the more important owing to the inherent difficulties in securing employer-sponsored schemes of insurance, more so in case of low-income rural residents. A study by the Urban Institute in the context of rural America documented that nearly a sixth (16%) of rural non-elderly people obtained insurance through state programs like Medicaid or the likes, compared to just over a tenth (11%) of urban residents. Rural people are already familiar with such public insurance programs and readily could avail the benefit of expanded public coverage[18].

4. Conclusion

Rural health insurance has been an effective means of saving poor rural people from having to make catastrophic healthcare payments. It can also contribute in improving rural livelihood in many other ways. Erstwhile evidence is suggestive of the feasibility of health insurance for the rural poor under certain conditions. Enhancing insurance coverage in rural areas can strengthen the system of healthcare a great deal. What is more important is that the socioeconomic situation of the rural poor may be influenced positively by health insurance. At that, the increase of the illness-induced financial risk and better healthcare access, indirect effects of rural health insurance like better health outcomes and increased labor productivity can materialize as well. The extent of health insurance or its absence thereof, largely influences people's willingness to agree to risky, but potentially beneficial investment needs further investigation. However, community structures do not necessarily ensure automatic and successful inclusion of the 'poorest of the poor'. Community participation can be inclusionary as well as exclusionary. This implies that certain characteristics of the community and design as well as implementation features of the schemes act as important determinants to achieve outcomes that are intended for rural poor. It is also necessary to be aware that

---

[18] National Rural Health Association, 1999, *op cit.*

community financing schemes cannot be considered as the sole solution to manage illness risks though they represent an important element. Based on some innovative practices, the governments can formulate policies so as to make it easier for rural families to get enrolled in public health insurance schemes.

Note: Inclusion of micro-insurance has been an enriching suggestion and it is incorporated accordingly. However, the second sub-heading does not have enough scope to be re-fragmented, and hence kept in its original form.

(Azmal Hussain, Consulting Editor, Icfai Research Centre, Kolkata. He can be reached at azmalhussain@icfai.org).

3

Chronic Disease Management Systems (Registries) in Rural Health Care

Anne Skinner, Roslyn Fraser-Maginn and Keith J Mueller

This article is focused on Chronic Disease Management Systems (CDMS), a tool that helps providers efficiently collect and analyze patient information to promote quality care for rural population. A CDMS is a patient-centered electronic database tool that helps providers diagnose, treat and manage chronic diseases. Citing evidences from the US, the authors point out that CDMS can be made really available to rural clinics and implemented as well as maintained by clinic staff with minimal technological expenditures. Health care providers can use CDMSs to capture and track scientific processes and outcome indicators related to the care of a patient diagnosed with a chronic disease. Finally, for an effective and sustainable change, implementation of CDMS should be accompanied by change in clinical processes, incorporation of interdisciplinary service and patients' participation.

Source: RUPRI, Center for Rural Health Policy Analysis (http:/www.unmc.edu/ruprihealth/Pubs/PB2006-1.pdf)

Purpose

Health care quality is being addressed from a variety of policy perspectives. The 2001 Institute of Medicine report, *Crossing the Quality Chasm*, calls for sweeping action involving a five-part strategy for change in the US health care system.[1] This agenda for change includes use of evidence-based approaches to address common conditions, the majority of which are chronic. A Chronic Disease Management System (CDMS), or registry, is a tool that helps providers efficiently collect and analyze patient information to promote quality care for the rural population. CDMSs can provide a technological entry point for the impending use of Electronic Medical Records.

A CDMS is a patient-centered electronic database tool that helps providers diagnose, treat, and manage chronic diseases. The purpose of this brief is to discuss the different types of CDMSs used by a sample of 14 state organizations and 19 local rural clinics in Maine, Nebraska, New Mexico, South Carolina, Washington, and Wisconsin.

As part of a larger study examining the challenges and innovations in implementing disease management programs in rural areas, we conducted interviews with national, state, and local contacts. During interviews, respondents helped us understand the usefulness and functionalities of commonly used CDMSs in rural facilities. Our focus was on the use of CDMSs in the management of diabetes, a disease prevalent in rural populations.

Key Findings

- CDMSs are readily available to rural clinics and are being implemented and maintained by clinic staff with minimal expenditures for technology.
- Use of a standardized system in a collaborative helps provide data comparisons and share costs involved with technical assistance services across the group.

Chronic Disease Management Systems

Health care providers use CDMSs to electronically capture and track specific processes and outcome indicators related to the care of a patient diagnosed with a chronic disease. A highly functional system is capable of the following:[2]

- Providing reminders at the point of care to prompt the care team to deliver recommended care.
- Generating exception reports that provide information about patients who are overdue for care or have clinical outcomes that indicate the chronic disease is not being managed effectively.
- Providing patients with graphs and charts of critical indicators to motivate and aid in self-management.
- Tracking facility-wide and provider performance consistent with evidence-based guidelines.
- Measuring the effectiveness of the clinic's disease management program through outcome indicators.
- Providing a record of care for communication across interdisciplinary teams and providers.
- Interfacing with the information systems of ancillary services such as laboratory and billing.

The following CDMSs were being used in rural diabetes management programs according to our interview respondents:

- Diabetes Electronic Management System (DEMS) and Chronic Disease Electronic Management System (CDEMS).
- Patient Electronic Care System (PECS).
- Program-sponsored CDMSs.
- Custom CDMSs.

Diabetes Electronic Management System and Chronic Disease Electronic Management System

Developed by the Washington State Diabetes Prevention and Control Program and released in 1999, DEMS was designed specifically to manage diabetes. An interview respondent offered the following background on DEMS:

"The Department of Health here, the Diabetes Prevention and Control Program, developed the registry that is used by the National Health Disparities Collaboratives

for community health centers, and so our state department here developed our own registry, and it continues on today. We have over 40,000 people in the registry.... Most of them have diabetes.... Over 100 clinics [participate]."

The Washington State Diabetes Prevention and Control Program released CDEMS in 2002 as a more flexible outgrowth of the DEMS system that customizes measures and incorporates other chronic diseases such as asthma, cardiovascular disease, and depression.

Both DEMS and CDEMS have the same basic functions, including the following:

- Store demographic information, visit dates and vitals, medications, diagnoses, services, labs, and notes.
- Produce reports of lab histories and graph selected measurements including lab results.
- Interface with selected laboratory systems.
- Generate patient-specific reports that can be used at the point of care to reinforce evidenced-based care.
- Provide reports to support patient self-management.
- Generate additional reports to measure provider and clinic compliance with recommended care indicators.

DEMS and CDEMS applications are available free of charge and require a PC with a Microsoft Windows 98 or later operating system. Microsoft Access, a database application included in the Microsoft Office Suite, is necessary to run the software, although working knowledge of the program is not required. In addition, users must have Internet access to download program files and upgrades and to receive technical assistance through the program Web site.

Clinics using DEMS or CDEMS benefited from the applications' ease of use and reporting capabilities. Collaborative groups were able to standardize reporting to compare results between facilities. Although it is possible, none of the clinics we spoke with had integrated any other ancillary systems, such as laboratory and billing, with DEMS or CDEMS. A user's group and technical support is provided through the CDEMS website.

Users' Perspectives of DEMS

> *"It [DEMS] is fantastic. I would absolutely hate it if I knew [they] were going to take this away from me."*

> *"The collaborative, this large quality improvement project [requires] that teams have a registry, a way of gathering population-based data. . . . They can choose any registry they want. CDEMS happens to be open source code, which means clinics can do anything they want to it. It's also free, free, free, free, free, and so is the technical assistance, so it makes it attractive."*

Patient Electronic Care System

Patient Electronic Care System, or PECS, is a software program developed by the Aristos Group in cooperation with the Bureau of Primary Health Care and the Institute for Health Care Improvement. The system was originally developed to specifically support the data needs of publicly funded community health centers participating in the National Health Disparities Collaboratives (HDCs). These collaboratives focus on patients with diabetes, cardiovascular disease, asthma, depression, cancer, and preventive service needs. PECS is modeled after the original registries (DEMS, CVDEMS [Cardiovascular and Diabetes Electronic Management System]) used in the beginning years of the collaborative program (see *http://www.pecsusers.net/about.asp*).

PECS has the same basic functions as DEMS. Unique PECS characteristics include the following:

- Facilities enter data and build reports through the Health Disparities National Reporting website (*www.HDNR.org*). This site is only available for participating facilities with a user name and password.
- Members gain the benefit of being able to access the reporting website to compare their results to those of other similar clinics.

PECS can be run on a stand-alone PC desktop with a Windows 2000 or later operating system. It can also be run through a client/server environment with Windows 98 SE or later, and the server on Windows NT4 sp5 or later and Microsoft SQL Server 7 or later. To access the reporting website, facilities must be able to connect to the Internet. At the time of our study, PECS was available free of charge only to clinics involved in an HDC. PECS is now available for purchase through the Aristos Group, Inc.

Respondents in our study indicated that belonging to the collaborative and using PECS is an advantage for chronic disease management programs at federally qualified health centers.

Users' Perspectives of PECS

"They [CHCs] do have Internet capabilities and certain programs that will be able to manage the PECS program. There will be some adjustments as far as the computer infrastructure. There are health centers that may have one computer at the front desk, so once they get into the Health Disparities Collaborative, they want the whole team to have e-mail and a computer. So there is some need to expand that."

"We also align them with this patient registry called PECS.... It [PECS] allows you to look at the measures and facilitate it with diabetes. So, for example, it may be that a patient comes into the clinic [who has] been diagnosed with diabetes and... the PECS system... says, 'Okay, you've got a patient with diabetes. Have they gotten the test for A1C? If they have received that test, did they get a second one within a certain amount of time?' The overarching... concept of this entire process of quality improvement or quality management is making sure that you are providing the services that [patients] need."

"Once they get set up, as you know, those registries are wonderful because of the materials they can extract and the way that they can practice... they can be so much more proactive. It's very helpful. It's worth all the time and grief in entering data. PECS will do graphs for you, such as all the diabetic patients within the last year or all of the A1Cs."

Program-Sponsored Chronic Disease Management Systems

Membership in a collaborative such as the HDC can help secure hardware, software, and support for technology. Some disease management programs recommend or require a specific CDMS. For example, the HDC requires that participants in their program have a CDMS and strongly recommends PECS. Having a standardized system facilitates sharing knowledge and comparing results against other program participants. Technical assistance through help lines, remote technical assistance, or on-site technical assistance is often provided free of charge for clinics using a program-sponsored CDMS.

The involvement of a Quality Improvement Organization (QIO) in a CDMS varies from state to state. No standard software program is required, recommended, or sponsored. A custom CDMS developed by one state QIO provides uniform data collection for clinics participating in quality improvement efforts. Participants send discs containing quarterly data downloaded from their PCs to the QIO for analysis. Data are compiled into reports that are shared with medical staff and then aggregated for comparison purposes. Use of the system is voluntary, and technical assistance is available with installation, implementation, and maintenance. Limited resources have prevented the QIO from providing the level of assistance desired, and they will no longer be starting clinics on the program.

"In terms of understanding, in the beginning... states were each developing their own [registry] and now there is some thought or discussion around adopting one more [registry] uniformly across all places. We, as a QIO, are thinking, do we push these clinics... to [use a QIO sponsored product] when in another 12 to 18 months, CMS is going to come down and say[they] have a better tool?"

Other QIOs view their collection of confidential CMS billing data and its subsequent analysis as a tool to determine if facilities and doctors are following specific clinical guidelines for the Medicare population. These data are beneficial for quality improvement guidelines, but the delay in reporting may not actually reflect what is currently happening.

"We do not collect that [patient data] directly from clinics. That data is their billing data that's actually submitted to CMS for reimbursement. That data is provided to QIOs to support the process of driving quality."

"Our data is updated quarterly, and we've got about a nine-month lag on the data, like what we have now with data was billed nine months ago.... But that's much better than it used to be.... It used to be a two-year lag time."

Asked whether the QIO relays info back to the clinic, one respondent answered as follows:

> *"We do, we definitely do, because we feel like not knowing is an awful thing. You need to know or there's no incentive to do anything if everybody can go merrily through their lives thinking, 'Oh we do great, oh yeah, every one of our patients, diabetic patients, get everything they need. I'm 100% at everything.' So we actually... mail a letter out.... We have a physician on staff who writes each doc.... We do a letter and we enclose each physician's own personal data so they can see that for themselves.... If they have any questions about it, they're welcome and invited to call our physician or one of our epidemiologists."*

State Physician-Hospital Organizations (PHOs) also have a stake in sharing data and improving quality within their region. A custom CDMS standardizes their data collection and provides the ability to give feedback to physicians to compare and improve their practices. Group collaboration also promotes cost-sharing of technical and administrative assistance.

> *"The registry is something that is really driven by the PHO. The PHO said, 'We're doing this.' So... 95% of the practices are doing it. And we're using that as a way to access the clinical data around participants in our program.... Anybody can enroll in different aspects of the diabetes care initiative here, and 95% of the practices are participating in the disease registry, so most of the people are covered."*

One state Medicaid program developed a diabetes disease registry system that uses claims and pharmacy data processed through an algorithm to determine persons who are clinically diagnosed with diabetes. The patient's claims are then examined to identify if certain diabetes quality measures are being met. If not, the practitioner and/or person with diabetes is notified. The system also aggregates data to determine individual facility guideline compliance compared to others in the state.

> *"What we will be doing is providing actual diabetic and some other chronic diseases expertise, really the latest cutting-edge care, talking to people in the clinics that participate in this initiative as well as providing a web-based registry*

for them to be able to be more proactive [in] population-based management of their diabetic patients.... Hopefully, we can move into other areas of chronic care... but our major focus will be... diabetic care. We are hoping to provide that to [state-level group] as a service... at no cost to them. We are in the planning stage of this."

"There's no sense in any practice having six or seven different registries, and the one that we'll be working with them on... can... integrate... most all the chronic diseases.... This company [is] headed up by a physician that's actually been working pretty closely with CMS folks... to develop a registry that CMS could then hand down to QIOs to hand down to physicians.... There's a couple of really good Web-based ones available, and DocSite seems to be an excellent system. We've done a lot of research into it; the cost is minimal, and we feel like we can help pick that up to get a good pilot going."

Custom Chronic Disease Management Systems

Small clinics can successfully build their own CDM, or registry, with spreadsheet and/or database software. Microsoft Office products such as Excel (spreadsheet software) and Access (database software) are popular choices for customized data tracking. Created by staff members who enjoy working with computers and data, applications range from simple to complex. Time consuming chart abstraction can be replaced by flexible data queries that allow for the monitoring and communication of quality improvement activities. Potential drawbacks to a custom registry are the lack of standardization for reporting and the inability to collaborate and benchmark with other facilities.

"The way we track is we have a special form of design, and our secretary... inputs [the data], and anytime I... want to know anything, I just ask her for that printout and... I know how many have had their hemoglobin A1C, or where they are with their classes, or whatever. So it's an in-house system that she [the secretary] formatted."

"The diabetes educators also have a registry in the Oracle database, and we created that as well. So they're able to track preimposed hemoglobin A1Cs and how many patients finish the program. There's a limited number [of measures]

that they gather, but they're able to look at how many patients at each of the centers are in the diabetes education program and how many haven't been through diabetes management education, and they do outreach to those patients... The only people who handle the educator's registry are the educators, and they fill out a sheet. It's really just like using DEMS. You have your encounter sheet, you make your checkmarks and fill in the info, and then it goes to someone for data entry."

Discussion

Rural clinics are beginning to feel increasing pressure to implement some type of electronic disease management system. Successful implementation, use, and sustainability of simple CDMSs have helped introduce technology into small rural clinics and have positively impacted chronic disease management programs.

Fear about the challenges of integrating data between CDMSs and electronic medical records could negatively influence the adoption rate of CDMSs. Facilities may choose to wait to implement any type of CDMSs in hopes of an all-encompassing system. Unfortunately, this delay could lead to data collection inefficiencies and stall quality improvement efforts that benefit from data accessibility and timely analysis.

"We [the state] are trying to implement some electronic medical records. One of our health centers already has Logician and several of the other health centers have decided that they are going to try Nexgen, and it is going to be phased in over a couple of years, so some are in the first phase and some are in the second phase. I think there are a total of eight health centers that will be implementing an electronic medical record in a year and a half to two years. A lot of people were hesitant. They said, 'If we're in the Health Disparities Collaborative and using PECS, then we won't be able to use EMR,' but it will transfer to PECS."

Finally, it is important to remember that a CDMS is just one component of an effective disease management strategy. Simply implementing an electronic disease management system without changing clinical processes, incorporating interdisciplinary services, and involving the patient will not lead to effective and sustainable change.

Acknowledgements

This project was funded by the Federal Office of Rural Health Policy, Health Resources and Services Administration, US Department of Health and Human Services, grant #1U1C RH03718.

(Anne Skinner has done her MSW from John Hopkins Bloomberg School of Public Health and associated with RUPRI;

Roslyn Fraser-Maginn, PhD and is now associated with RUPRI; and

Keith J Mueller is a Professor and the Director of the RUPRI Center for Rural Health Policy Analysis at the University of Nebraska Medical Center.)

4

A Web-Based Graphical User Interface for Evidence-Based Decision-Making for Health Care Allocations in Rural Areas

Nadine Schuurman, Margo Leight and Myriam Berube

Background: ***The creation of successful health policy and location of resources increasingly relies on evidence-based decision-making. The development of intuitive, accessible tools to analyse, display and disseminate spatial data potentially provides the basis for sound policy and resource allocation decisions. As health services are rationalized, the development of tools such as Graphical User Interfaces (GUIs) is especially valuable as they assist decision-makers in allocating resources such that the maximum number of people are served. GIS can be used to develop GUIs that enable spatial decision-making.***

Results: ***We have created a Web-based GUI (wGUI) to assist health policy-makers and administrators in the Canadian province of British Columbia make well-informed***

Source: International Journal of Health Geographics 2008, 7:49 (www.ij-healthgeographics.com/content/7/1/49).

decisions about the location and allocation of time-sensitive service capacities in rural regions of the province. This tool integrates datasets for existing hospitals and services, regional populations and road networks to allow users to ascertain the percentage of population in any given service catchment who are served by a specific health service, or baskets of linked services. The wGUI allows policy-makers to map trauma and obstetric services against rural populations within pre-specified travel distances, illustrating service capacity by region.

Conclusion: The wGUI can be used by health policy makers and administrators with little or no formal GIS training to visualize multiple health resource allocation scenarios. The GUI is poised to become a critical decision-making tool especially as evidence is increasingly required for distribution of health services.

Background

The Move to Evidence-Based Public Policy

Policy-makers are increasingly recognizing the importance of evidence-based decision-making – based on integrating results from the best available systematic research with seasoned professional judgment and expertise. Evidence-Based Decision-Making (EBDM) requires a commitment of resources to support the identification of pertinent questions and the research initiatives most appropriate to answer them. For issues requiring broad-based consultation with constituents and federal-provincial partnerships, this approach ensures that a defensible assessment methodology, based on the best available evidence, is brought to bear in supporting the choice of policy or program [1-5].

The benefits to health policy of EBDM are many: greater consistency in decision-making; a stronger likelihood of improved health outcomes from decisions based on reputable evidence; the potential for more cost-effective solutions with supporting evidence; program performance monitoring criteria that allow comparison with other programs; and the opportunity for further learning from experience [2,3,5-7].

Spatial Decision Support Systems (SDSS) as an Aid to Evidence-Based Policy-Making

Geographic Information Systems (GIS) offer a suite of spatial tools and methods that allow the user to analyze the spatial dimensions of health service location. GIS can be used to map sites, as well as build scenarios of different service arrangements. It is a particularly useful application for understanding the spatial dimensions of health care service delivery, and in particular the relationship between health outcomes and accessibility [8,9]. In many instances, GIS has been used to plan health care service delivery models as well as the optimal arrangement of health care facilities [10]. In order to execute these analyses, however, the ability to link health care services (hospitals) with potential patients is required.

GIS is a component of many Decision Support Systems (DSS), which range from DSS generators to the latest flexible modelling tools based on query systems, spreadsheets, statistical software packages and GIS programs. DSS tools include powerful modelling functions; data streamlining capabilities and management features to access internal and external data; analytical capabilities and visual representations of relationships; and powerful but simple user interfaces [11,12]. Decision-making problems with a large number of decision alternatives and outcomes that vary spatially require Spatial Decision Support Systems (SDSS) with large data management and integration capacity [13-16]. Geographic location can be the key feature in making data meaningful for decision-makers by linking different datasets by their spatial commonalities [17]. Prior to accessible GIS tools, considering the relationship between factors influencing a decision, for example whether to close a hospital ward, was a mathematical and economic modelling exercise with limited opportunity for the decision-makers to rework scenarios after the problem was defined [18].

Making SDSS Accessible in Health Services Policy: Employing a Web-Based Graphical User Interface (wGUI)

A Graphical User Interface (GUI) designed to reduce cognitive load through a more structured presentation of strategic information can increase the comfort level with decision-making activities. User-supportive GUI design results in a wider deliberation of options [19] through reduced data framing bias [20,21];

more successful concept communication [22,23]; and ease of user-constructed scenarios [24-26]. Decision-makers explore relationships that are otherwise obscure when the decision-maker is in control of the scenario generation [19,27]. The lower costs of a Web-based GUI (wGUI) supported by SDSS can increase the stakeholder involvement in health service policy-making by reducing the facilitation and planning time needed to address a specific issue [12,13,20,28].

GIS support for evidence-based health policy decision-making has been constrained by reliance on GIS specialists, limiting the opportunity for considering all possible decision outcomes [1,25,29]. GIS must continue to perform traditional functions, but the training expense, time commitment, and cost of equipment with suitable software are often barriers for users [30-32]. Removing barriers to wide scale adoption of GIS as a decision-making tool requires reduced training requirements, intuitive use of the software platforms and low cost access to information. If human-factor guidelines are considered, i.e., "users' platform-independent access to georegistered data, meta-data, and other related information via a windows, icon, mouse...user interface" [27], the use of the Internet becomes a desirable venue.

The development of a Web-based SDSS tool is consistent with current global changes in the Web. Web 2.0 broadly refers to a new generation of Internet services and technology. This *second wave* of the World Wide Web [33] has revolutionized communication via the Internet just as the original Web revolutionized information dissemination and access. Web 2.0 promises to democratize the Internet in a way not seen before and to a large degree this is being achieved through participation amongst Web users [34, 35]. The goal of Web 2.0 is a richer, more complete Web experience available to all Internet users. While there is debate over what Web 2.0 truly comprises, several key themes have emerged as the term has entered widespread use. 'The participatory Web' as opposed to 'the Web as information source' is frequently attached to descriptions of Web 2.0, of which user-created content and collaboration are the hallmarks. In fact, the idea that the average Internet user can create content is considered an essential element of Web 2.0 [36]. In comparison with the previous iteration of the Web, the new Web encourages significantly more interaction between users [37]. In addition, open access and open source are important themes for Web 2.0 [38].

The term Web 2.0 is more than just a paradigm for describing different patterns of usage; it is also a technology paradigm [39]. A key theme of Web 2.0 is the 'Internet as platform.' Cheung *et al.* [40] outline the applications that define Web 2.0: *rich Internet applications, collaboration tools, user contributed content databases, and integrative technologies.* The advent of Web-based applications promises to reduce the dominance of proprietary software manufacturers, as these tools are often free or are at least provided at a significantly reduced cost compared with their traditional desktop counterparts. Given the rapid shift of the Web to a highly socialized, interactive environment, it is inevitable that SDSS will migrate to the Web as the platform of choice. The wGUI is a preliminary instantiation of the Web 2.0.

Web applications such as a wGUI can support cross-platform analysis and data sharing among decision-making groups of diverse technical skills and physical locations [33]. Access to shared information is possible at any time and place with minimal infrastructure supports through client-server architecture. Web client programs (browsers) are relatively simple to use because document mark-up language ensures consistent information presentation across individual hardware and software platforms. Decision-makers are accustomed to pervasive browsers and no additional training or software maintenance is required to support their use of this venue for SDSS delivery. A wGUI is an innovative means of using Web 2.0 technologies to facilitate evidence-based health policy decision-making.

A New Approach to Health Policy-making

Employing a wGUI to Facilitate Health Policy-making

The drive to more inclusive decision-making in health care policy and procedural processes has challenged the expert community to develop venues for rapidly informing decision-makers. Not only must information be readily available, there is a need to inform non-expert decision-makers of the relevance of different information and how the data has informed past decisions. One of the means of providing distributed decision-makers with differing expertise with a common framework for decision-making is a wGUI. In this instance, the data retrieval, analysis and processing for the wGUI is provided by a Web-enabled GIS tool that incorporates an expert understanding of the problem and a range of solution sets. Adjectives describing a good user interface include consistent, comprehensible, natural, responsive, self-explanatory, efficient, flexible, effective, and rewarding.

Bhargava, Power *et al.*, broadly classify a wide range of customized and generic DSS into five families of DSS tools. Data driven DSS organize, analyse and retrieve large volumes of data using database queries and use online analytical processing (OLAP) techniques. Model-driven DSS represent decision models and through analysis, optimization, stochastic modeling, simulation, statistics and logic modeling, provide analysis support. Web interfaces have expanded the DSS applications to open ended problems with fuzzier choices in the form of three other types of DSS that have now become widespread. Communication driven DSS link multiple decision-makers over space and time. Knowledge driven DSS assist with selection of alternatives, such as medical expert systems and scenario generators. Document driven DSS integrate a variety of storage and processing technologies to provide document retrieval and analysis {Bhargava, 2007 #299}.

In 1995 Jones [34] identified the seamless integration of user interface and DSS functionality as a key development in DSS. User interface had been a secondary consideration with the widely used data driven and model driven DSS tools. SDSS adoption research, however, challenges the idea that user satisfaction with Web-enabled DSS tools is primarily related to systems and information quality [12,23,28,35-38]. Rather, studies have shown that SDSS users experienced self-efficacy gains when working with user interface features that prioritized information presentation, resulting in perceived efficiency and decision quality improvements. The time-and-effort savings of an intuitively designed user interface mitigate a perspective that SDSS may take too much time and effort to use [24,26,39].

Once the need for a wGUI is established, it is important to ensure simple and clean design to maximize the user potential. Elvins and Jain summarize the factors of good GUI design and support the increasing use of wGUI [27]. One of the goals of wGUI for SDSS is minimizing the need for GIS technical knowledge. Well-designed user interfaces adopt a conceptual model that is familiar, and incorporate easy to understand and appropriate visual metaphors with a simple and uncluttered layout. An important feature of the wGUI is being accessible to users with varying abilities through the provision of interactive help functions. There is always the option, as the users become more adept, of turning off these functions. A well-structured user interface will minimize the amount of user work-arounds or problem solving.

An illustration of how a wGUI could address the expert concerns is found in a review of a collection of SDSS tools for integrated coastal management that involves marine, estuarine, wetland and coastal systems in topical areas. The adoption of SDSS tools – the key points of success are the involvement of the end user in the development of the tools, design for end-user needs, a flexible adaptive and updatable system with an easy to use interface that requires limited time invested to learn the system {West-macott, 2001 #311}.

Execution of tasks using SDSS – and their results – need to be reliably predictable. This is especially true when there are several ways to achieve the same results. A wGUI limits the possible ways of working with SDSS and as a consequence, reduces the number of ways it can produce incorrect results. User errors will still occur but it is easier to address these when they do if there are limitations on what modifications to the SDSS and data sources are possible.

Optimal Location and Ensuring Maximum Access to Health Services: Creating a wGUI to Facilitate Health Services Location

In response to the specific needs of health policy within British Columbia, we have developed a wGUI designed to assist BC health policy-makers in making better informed decisions about service reallocations and hospital closures or openings affecting rural regions in BC. Potential users of this wGUI include *British Columbia Ministry of Health* Medical Officers and Information Officers who are charged with making decisions about service provision. A number of allocation decisions are devolved to the level of the regional Health Authority; thus the five Health Authorities in the province are also likely users.

The wGUI is designed to provide information about the geographical extent of service catchments around health services in rural and remote British Columbia (e.g., the entire province excluding the two metropolitan areas of Victoria and Vancouver). A catchment is a designated geographical area around a service. In addition, the wGUI provides information about the total number of people in each existing or hypothetical service catchment as well as percentages of the population *not served* within the specified road travel time.

In this case, the catchment sizes were defined as one, two and four hour drive times. These designations reflect the standards set by the *British Columbia Ministry of Health* specifying the maximum acceptable distances to any given health service. The provincial standards specify, for instance, that access to emergency services (24/7/52) should be provided within a one hour travel time for 98% of the population [48]. Likewise, access to basic inpatient hospital services should be within two hours travel time for 98% of the population [48]. Finally, the province's standards of accessibility for services specify that core specialty services should be available within four hours travel time for 98% of residents [48]. There is evidence that time to definitive care is an important factor in outcome. In the case of trauma, for example, research has indicated that access to service within the "golden hour" has a profound positive effect on outcome [49,50].

Using the wGUI, planners can determine the extent to which the province is fulfilling its own mandate for service provision to 98% of the population within specified travel times for specific services. The wGUI can also be used to support decisions about hospital closures, openings and service reallocations in rural and remote regions in BC – as it provides numbers of people served for a given health service within specified times. The wGUI is designed to allow health planners and administrators to determine the optimal location of health services based primarily on the criterion of serving the largest possible population within certain road travel time catchments.

The initial version of the wGUI illustrated here allows catchment calculation and associated population reporting for regional and provincial levels of trauma and maternity services throughout the province of British Columbia. In addition, it allows health policy planners to analyse scenarios for *all* hospitals in British Columbia – without specific service differentiation.

At present, the wGUI incorporates detailed service data for trauma and maternity services – though more service baskets are currently being added. In addition, it excludes the two Central Metropolitan Areas (CMAs) of Vancouver and Victoria as there is considerable overlap between services in urban areas so access in these regions is a less pressing issue.

Results

The wGUI we have developed was created to enable health policy-makers and administrators in BC to generate evidence to support their decision-making process, specifically about the location and allocation of time-sensitive service capacities in rural regions of the province. It was designed to facilitate use by a broad group of stakeholders with varying levels of expertise across a range of locations.

When the wGUI is launched, the opening screen reveals seven screens. The lower left screen illustrated in Figure 1 allows the user to choose a maximum travel time, a Health Authority and a set of hospitals. The Maximum Travel Time options are one hour, two hours or four hours while the Health Authority options comprise BC's provincial health regions: Fraser, Interior, Northern, Vancouver Coastal, Vancouver Island and "All BC". The central screen in the main window contains a map of British Columbia divided into the five Health Authorities (i.e., the chief administrative planning bodies), showing all the roads and hospitals in the province (Figure 1). Users may select a set of BC hospitals, by name or services offered, and determine the number of people in a particular Health Authority (or all of BC) within a specified travel time of each hospital. The resultant analysis

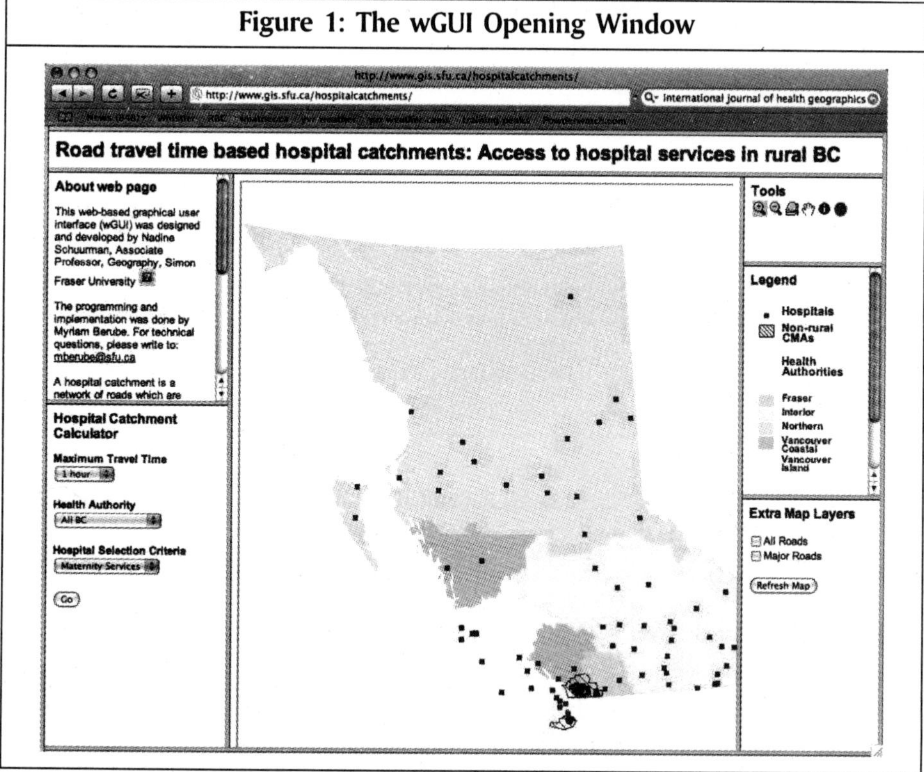

Figure 1: The wGUI Opening Window

will illustrate the number of people served and conversely those excluded from services within the travel time defined for the scenario. Users may also run analyses with hospitals added or removed from the initial selection – in order to visualize effects of health services closures or openings. They can then compare the populations served within hospital catchments before and after each change.

The subsequent wGUI window depends on the user's hospital selection criterion. For example, if the user selected a two hour maximum travel time for trauma services in the Northern Health Authority (as illustrated in Figure 2), then a new window illustrated in Figure 3 would open allowing the user to refine the basket of trauma services selected. The trauma services choices are consistent with level one (tertiary), level two (regional) and level three (basic) services.

Figure 2: Choosing Trauma Service Catchment Parameters

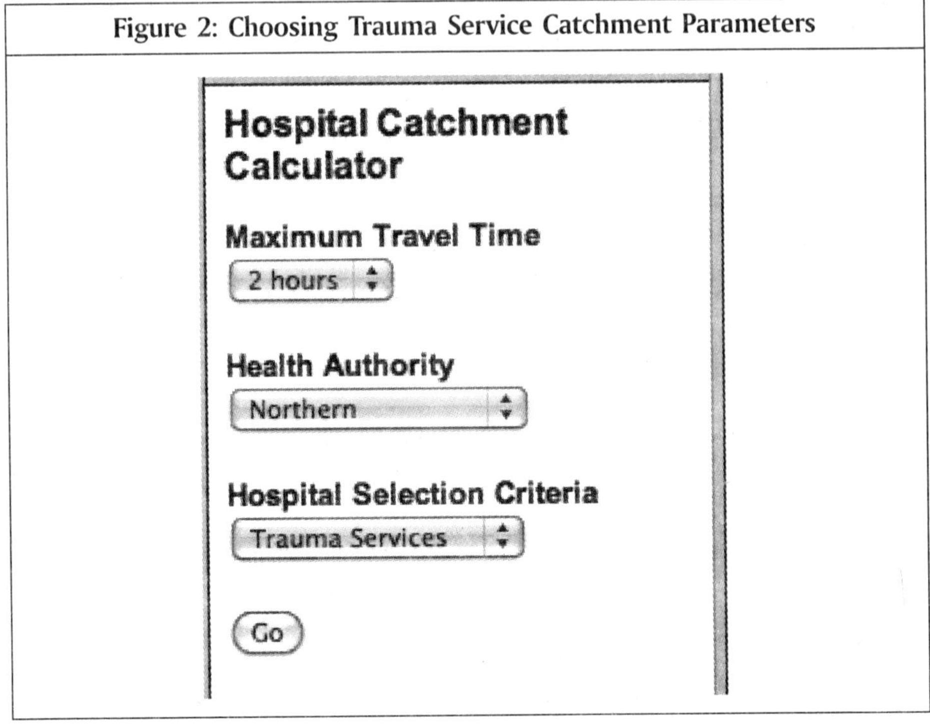

Alternatively, if maternity services were chosen, a window with options for levels of maternity service from midwife to full obstetrical services follows. In each case, the user is presented with a list of hospitals that fit that service criteria as well as a second list that enables them to model alternate scenarios in which

Figure 3: Choosing Trauma Service Levels

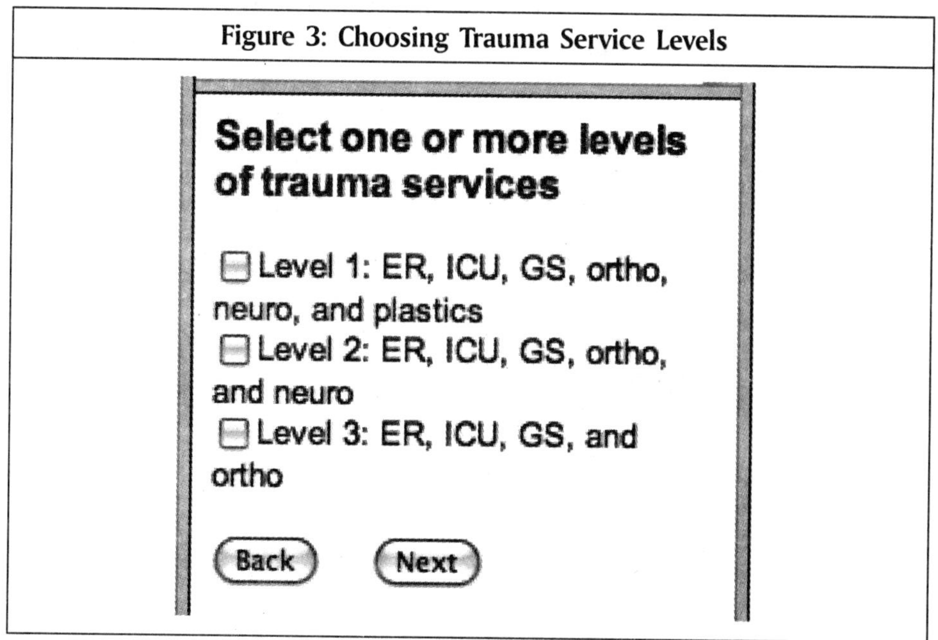

hospital services are added. The user can choose to delete a hospital from the top list of those that fulfil the service criteria to determine what percentage of the population would be adversely affected by service removal. These choices are illustrated in Figure 4.

When "Next" is selected in the Figure 4 window, a "View Catchment Report" button is presented. When that button is clicked, an html page opens in the user's Web browser with a table displaying the hospitals which satisfy the user's choices. The resulting table from this sample catchment calculation is illustrated in Figure 5.

In addition, a map of the catchment around the selected hospital(s) is drawn in the central wGUI screen – as illustrated in Figure 6.

The wGUI allows the user to select British Columbia hospitals by name or services offered, as well as by travel time from populations anywhere in British Columbia or within a specific Health Authority. Moreover, users can modify the list of suitable hospitals by removing or adding hospitals to simulate the closure or addition of services. The wGUI creates a table with the final list of hospitals

Figure 4: The list of hospitals with the selected trauma service level – as well as other BC hospitals. The latter list can be used to select additional hospitals where policy-makers may want to model added services to determine the effect on numbers of people served within the selected two hour travel time catchment

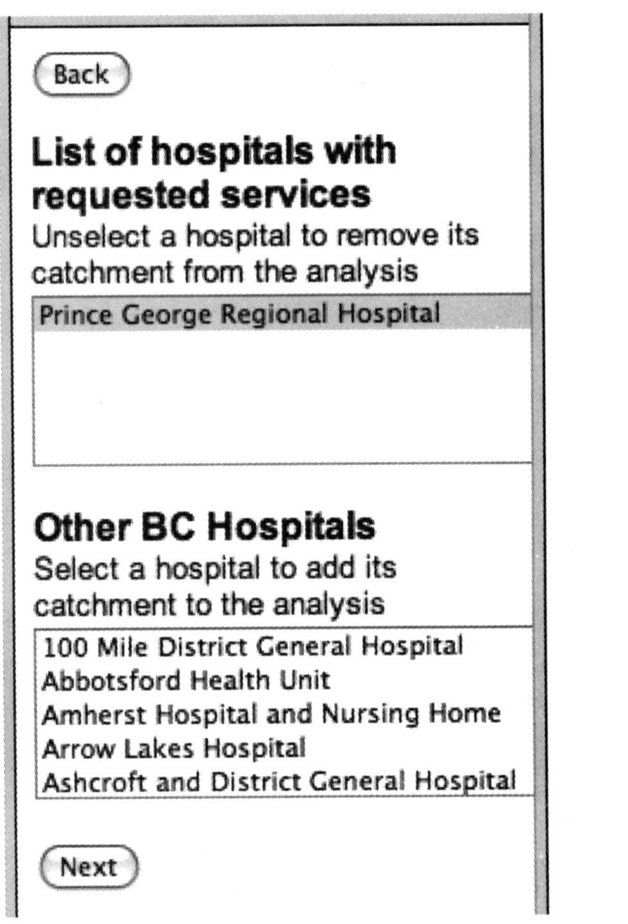

and the populations within the chosen travel time and health authority. The table also lists the populations within the chosen Health Authority (or all BC) that are outside the hospital catchments. If there are populations that live within the chosen travel time of more than one suitable hospital, they are assigned to the closest one. The wGUI adds graphical representations of the hospital catchments

Figure 5: The table generated with the "View Catchment Report" button is pressed. This table illustrates the total population served within the two hour catchment travel time for the selected service in the selected Health Authority. In this case, 41.36% of the population of the extensive Northern Health Authority is *not served* within two hours travel time of the most basic level 3 trauma services. This report communicates important information about the vulnerability of rural and remote populations and serves to inform administrators of where health services may be needed

Hospital Catchments

Rural population/area of interest: Northern Health Authority
Maximum gravel time: 2 hours
Service Type: trauma
Level: 3
Hospitals removed:

Hospital ID	Hospital Name	Rural Population Served	Percent of Northern Rural Population
93	Prince George Regional Hospital	117,861	41.36
Total rural population served		117,861	41.36
Rural population not served		167,128	58.64
Northern Rural Population		284,989	100

to a map of British Columbia. The user can zoom in, zoom out and pan the map, as well as get hospital information by clicking on a hospital square. Figure 7 illustrates the application flow and describes the underlying algorithmic processes.

The wGUI is built on a foundational ArcMap GUI. The latter refreshes the map image more quickly and allows the user to perform further analysis on the hospital catchment features by using the many ArcMap tools and by adding other data to the map. However, it also requires an expensive ArcGIS Desktop license and some knowledge of GIS software. The functionality of the wGUI may be more limited but anyone with a password and a Web browser can use it and additional functionality will be added in the future as the GUI is developed.

Discussion

There are a number of benefits to developing a wGUI for policy-makers and health administrators to use in allocating resources in rural and remote areas where

Figure 6: The catchment map generated by the sample query. In the case the catchment – shown in orange – represents a two hour road travel time from Prince George Regional Hospital in British Columbia's Northern Health Authority (NHA). Prince George is the only hospital to offer any trauma services in the NHA

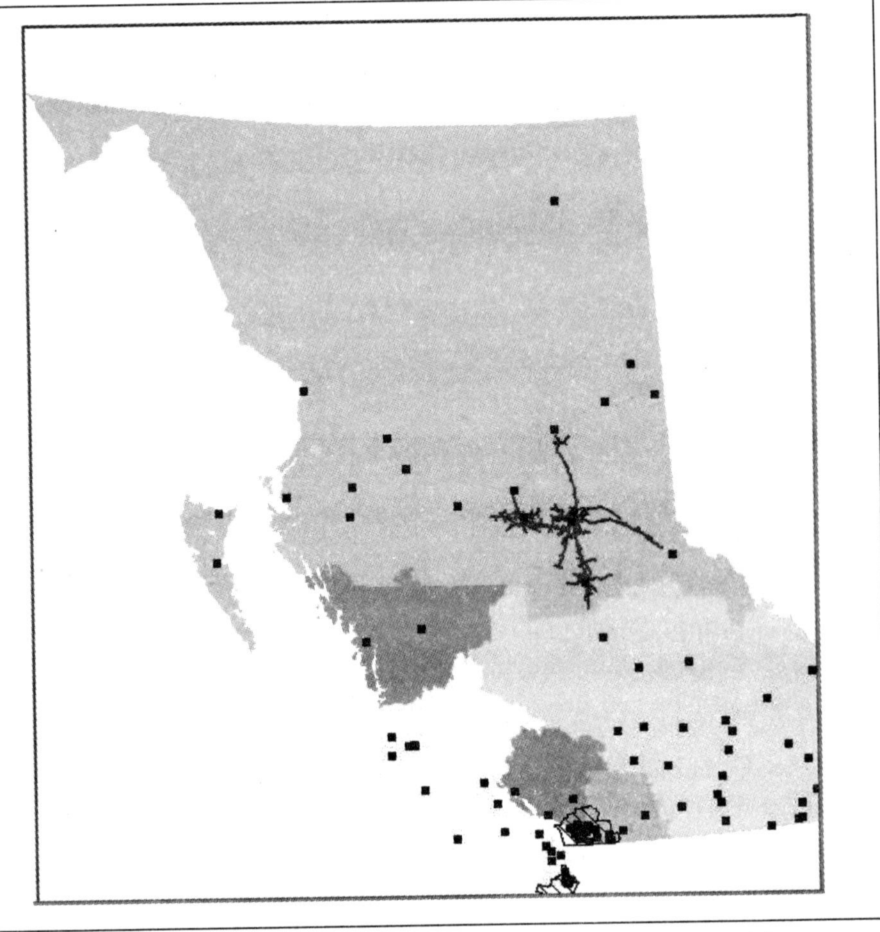

catchments seldom overlap – especially given their constrained financial resources. The wGUI is readily accessible from the Web, requires no expertise in spatial analysis, and is easy to use. It delivers clear results in map form as well as providing the population figures needed to support decisions about allocation that will benefit the greatest numbers of people. In a policy environment that is increasingly espousing the value of evidence-based decision-making, such tools are especially important.

Figure 7: The wGUI presents the user with a series of choices in order to direct their query. The user steps are summarized in this flowchart and underlying processing is explained for each step

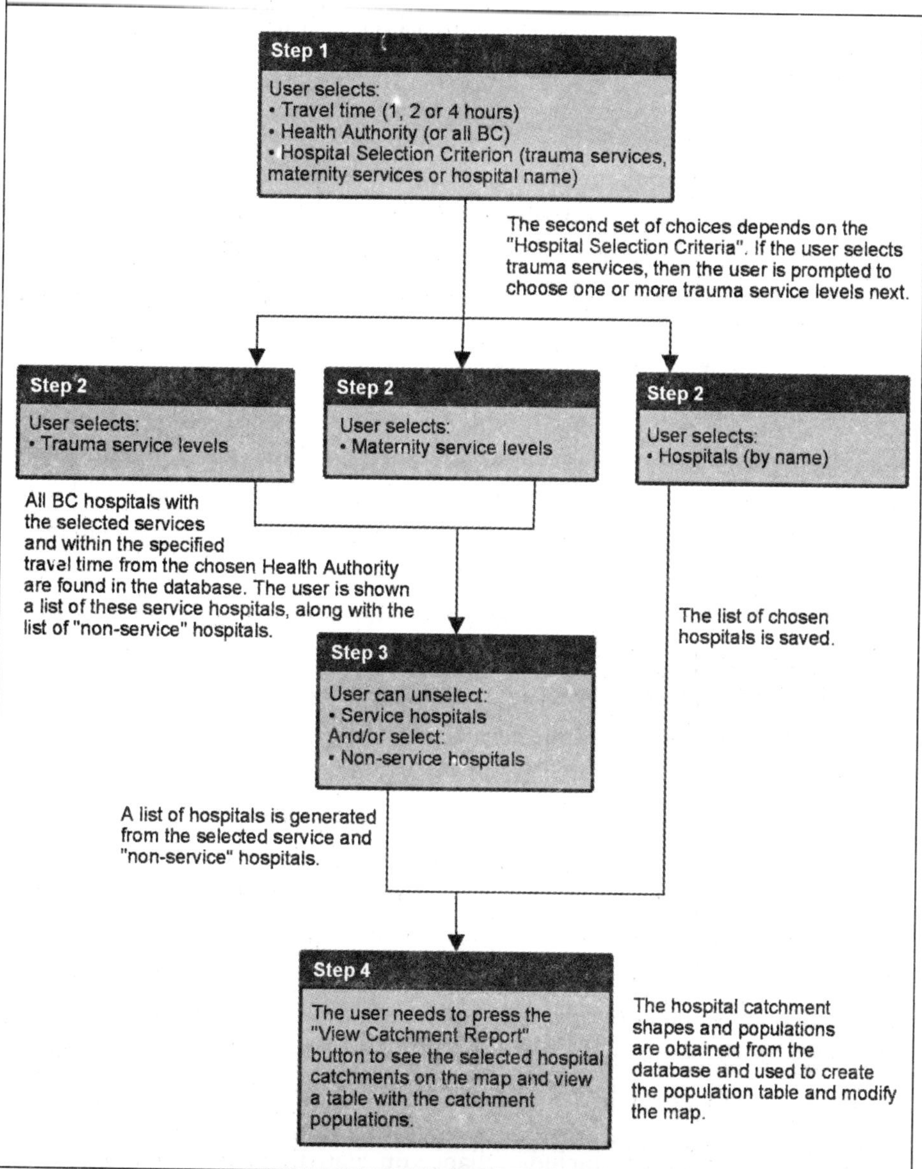

In the Canadian province of British Columbia where mountainous regions constrain car travel, incorporating travel time calculations into the wGUI to determine level of access imbues the results with greater reliability. This is especially pertinent as fewer than 7% of traumatic injuries, for example, are airlifted from rural and remote areas. We expect that the wGUI will prove useful in other rural and remote jurisdictions nationally and generally provide a critical addition to support evidence-based decision-making for health care.

Decision-making tools need to be designed so they do not integrate hidden errors and thereby facilitate faulty interpretation [51]. There is a risk that a Web-based SDSS tool might allow users lacking in GIS skills to draw the wrong conclusions, leading to non-rational decisions. Ideally, a user should only be able to produce valid results and maps. In this case, the wGUI is not designed to operate as a decision-making framework and is therefore not providing information subject to interpretation. It serves as a check against population access to health services within mandated road travel time, returning information on the spatial extent of one, two and four hour road travel time catchments. In addition, it provides supporting tables that illustrate the percentages of total population served and not served within the query region. The nature of information rendered, therefore, does not allow for misinterpretation. Should wGUIs based on GIS become more prevalent, it will be important to ensure that they are designed to prevent users without broad spatial awareness from reaching the wrong conclusions.

Limitations

Perhaps the most obvious limitation to the wGUI is the fact that many health allocation decisions are made based on a large number of internal and political pressures that are unrelated to evidence. Many decisions are made independent of rational evidence with respect to resource allocation. Indeed, there is evidence that models are sometimes used only to buttress decisions – once they are already made [52]. Perhaps the greatest danger is not lack of evidence-based policy but the generation of policy-based evidence [52].

Additional limitations include reliance on Statistics Canada population data which, although quite accurate, is collected only every five years. Also, at present, only two specific health services (trauma and maternity) are included in the model though our group intends to add cardiac, ER, palliative and oncology services shortly.

Conclusion

The wGUI described in this paper was constructed specifically to aid hospital administrators and health policy-makers in making decisions about allocation of resources. The wGUI is accessible to users with little or no GIS experience and is easy to use over the Web. It permits users to visualize the geographical area served by a specific hospital service such as trauma or rural maternity. In addition, it provides accurate population estimates of people served within a one, two or four hour travel time from a specific hospital service. Finally, the wGUI enables policy-makers to create scenarios in which a hospital is added or removed – and visualize the resulting impact on the population served. This tool is poised to become an integral component of evidence-based decision-making for the allocation of health services when the goal is to serve the maximum number of people in dispersed rural and remote regions.

Methods

Data

Five datasets were used to develop the GUI: BC hospital data, BC road network data, BC census block population data, BC Health Authority data and BC Census Metropolitan Area data. The hospital data included attributes indicating the presence or absence of various health services (e.g., neurosurgery; ICU). The road features were associated with vehicle travel times for both directions. The census block centroid point features linked to population values were used to determine populations within specific travel times of a hospital. BC Health Authority polygons allow the option of permitting the user to restrict analysis to particular Health Authorities. Finally, the BC Census Metropolitan Areas (CMAs) were used to restrict the analysis to rural areas of BC, by masking the Vancouver and Victoria CMAs.

Five new datasets were derived from the five datasets listed above: an origin-destination cost table, a Health Authority population table and 3 hospital catchment feature classes for one, two and four hour travel times.

The data used by the ArcMap GUI was stored in an Access geodatabase. When the wGUI was created, this data was copied to an Oracle database to allow concurrent multiuser access. An ArcSDE Server was used as the gateway between the GIS software and the Oracle database.

GUI Construction

Creating the Road Network Dataset

ESRI's ArcCatalog 9.1 and Network Analyst tools were used to create a geodatabase road network dataset. Before building this network dataset, attributes were added for travel time in each direction along a road segment. To calculate these times, the segment length, speed limit and presence of a stop sign or light were considered. Stop signs were assumed to add 30 seconds to the travel time while lights were assumed to add one minute. Some road features were also removed prior to network dataset creation. Road features with a road classification of lane, ferry or trail were removed. Roads in the non-rural Central Metropolitan Areas (CMAs) that provide the fastest access to each non-rural hospital from rural areas were identified. All other roads in the non-rural regions were removed to decrease the density of the road network in this region and thus speed up network analysis involving non-rural hospitals.

Creating the Origin-Destination Cost Table

ESRI's Network Analyst New OD Cost Matrix tool (in Arc-Map 9.1) was used to create the origin-destination cost table. The BC hospital points were loaded as destinations and the rural BC census block centroid points within 2.5 kilometres of a road were loaded as origins. Travel times less than 4 hours were calculated for all hospital and centroid (within 2.5 kilometres) combinations. Fields for census block population, census block health authority, hospital maternity service level and hospital trauma service level were added to the table created by the New OD Cost Matrix tool.

Creating the Hospital Catchment Feature Classes

Hospital catchments, or service areas, were created in Arc-Map 9.1 using the Network Analyst New Service Area tool. This process required hospital point features as well as a road network dataset. For each maximum travel time (one, two and four hours), a feature class composed of road line networks around each hospital was generated. Hospital catchments that were distributed across more than one health authority were split along the health authority boundaries. Thus, the wGUI can select catchments by hospital and health authority.

Creating the ArcMap GUI

Visual Basic for Applications, or VBA, is an embedded programming environment that can be used to automate, customize and extend ESRI applications such as ArcMap. Before developing the wGUI, we decided to build the GUI as an ArcMap macro using ScenarioBuilder, in order to develop and test the data and code required for the GUI. ScenarioBuilder allowed the creation of various pop-up windows that permit the user to select hospital catchment analysis options. It also adds catchment features to an Arc-Map document map already showing BC hospitals, health authorities and roads.

Porting the GUI to the Web

The ArcMap version of the GUI (described above) can only be utilized by users with ArcGIS Desktop (software which includes the ArcMap application) installed on their personal computer. The data required for the hospital catchment maps and calculations must also be located on the user's computer, clearly limiting functionality for the vast majority of potential users.

To create a Web GUI with an interactive map of British Columbia's hospitals and roads, a software application for publishing interactive maps on the Internet was required. ESRI's ArcIMS 9.1 software was used to perform this task. Furthermore, a Web server was needed to serve the Website; a coding language for developing the Web application had to be selected; and the data needed to be stored in a database which allows concurrent access to one data layer by multiple users.

The ArcIMS software was installed on a machine running an Apache HTTP Server. Since many of the ArcIMS components were built with Java, a Java Development Kit (JDK) and a servlet engine (Apache Tomcat) also needed to be installed.

It is possible to create a Website using an ArcIMS template but this requires using javascript and ArcXML to add functionality. Since creating the Hospital Catchment Web GUI involved coding a great deal of custom functionality, it was decided to create a custom Web application using Java Server Pages. Thus, the Java Connector, which contains the ArcIMS Java Connector API JavaBeans, was installed with ArcIMS. These JavaBeans and their methods can be used in Java code to implement map related functions. The ArcSDE Java API JavaBeans were also used to query the tables in the Oracle database. The ArcSDE Java API was obtained from the ArcSDE Client software. The data were copied to an Oracle database, which allows concurrent multi-user access and an ArcSDE server functioned as the gateway between the database and the GIS software.

To create the hospital and population table reports (illustrated in Figures 5, and 6), ActiveX Data Objects (ADO) and SQL were used in the VBA code to query the origin-destination cost table. The query picks all the records in the origin-destination cost table with the hospital names, maternity service levels, trauma service levels, health authority, and travel time chosen by the user. If a census block occurs more than once in all the records that satisfy the user's selections, only the record with the lowest travel time is chosen (note that more than one hospital can be less than the maximum travel time from a census block centroid). For each hospital, the census block populations are summed. The total rural population of the chosen Health Authority is taken from the HAPopulations table. If the user is interested in all rural BCPopulations, the population values in the HAPopulations table are summed. ArcObjects is used in the VBA code to select the catchments from the travel time appropriate Hospital Catchments feature class (one, two or four hours).

Competing Interests

The authors declare that they have no competing interests.

Authors' Contributions

NS conceptualized the study, designed the methodology, secured the data, supervised the GUI and wGUI development and wrote and revised this paper. ML researched other GUI work and spatial decision support systems. MB prepared the data, developed and implemented the Arc-GIS and Web GUIs. In addition, she tested the prototypes. All authors read and approved the final manuscript.

Acknowledgements

The authors would like to thank the Canadian Institutes for Health Research (CIHR) Grant #149353 as well as Michael Smith Foundation for Health Research for invaluable assistance in developing this application and providing the time to do so. Also thanks to Ellen Randall for carefully reviewing several drafts of this paper.

(Nadine Schuurman, Corresponding author, Department of Geography, Simon Fraser University, Burnaby, Canada. The author can be reached at nadine@sfu.ca

Margo Leight, Computer Science, Simon Fraser University, Burnaby, Canada. The author can be reached at guertin@cs.sfu.ca; and

Myriam Berube, Department of Geography, Simon Fraser University, Burnaby, Canada. The author can be reached at mberube@sfu.ca).

References

1. Boulos MNK: Towards evidence-based, GIS-driven national spatial health information infrastructure and surveillance services in the United Kingdom. *International Journal of Health Geographics* 2004, 3:1-50.
2. Gagnon F, Turgeon J, Dallaire C: Healthy public policy: A conceptual cognitive framework. *Health Policy* 2007, 81:42-55.
3. Hausman AJ: Implications of Evidence-based Practice for Community Health. *American Journal of Community Psychology* 2002, 30:453-467.
4. Hewison A: Evidence-based management in the NHS: is it possible? *Journal of Health Organisation and Management* 2004, 18:336-348.
5. Sanderson I: Making Sense of 'What Works': Evidence-based Policy-making as Instrumental Rationality? *Public Policy and Administration* 2002, 17:61-75.
6. Fulcher CL, Kaukinen CE: Visualizing the infrastructure of US healthcare using Internet GIS: a community health informatics approach for reducing health disparities. *Stud Health Technol Inform* 2004, 107 (Pt 2):1197-1201.
7. Sanderson I: Evaluation, Policy Learning and Evidence-Based Policy-making. *Public Administration* 2002, 80:1-22.
8. McLafferty SL: GIS and Health Care. *Annual Review of Public Health* 2003, 24:25-42.
9. Schuurman N, Fiedler RS, Grzybowski SC, Grund D: Defining rational hospital catchments for non-urban areas based on travel-time. *International Journal of Health Geographics* 2006, 5.

10. Gatrell A, Senior M: Health and health care applications. In *Geographical Information Systems: Principles, Techniques, Management and Applications 2nd Abridged edition* Edited by: Longley PA, Goodchild MF, Maguire DJ, Rhind DW. New York: John Wiley & Sons; 2005.
11. Bhargava HK, Sridhar S, Herrick C: Beyond Spreadsheets: Tools for Building Decision Support Systems. *IEEE Computer* 1999, 32:31-39.
12. Shim JP, Warkentin M, Courtney JF, Power DJ, Sharda R, Carlsson C: Past, present, and future of decision support technology. *Decision Support Systems* 2002, 33:111-126.
13. Westmacott S: Developing decision support systems for integrated coastal management in the tropics: Is the ICM decision-making environment too complex for the development of a useable and useful DSS? *Journal of Environmental Management* 2001, 62:55-74.
14. Higgs G: A Literature Review of the Use of GIS-Based Measures of Access to Health Care Services. *Health Services and Outcomes Research Methodology* 2004, 5.
15. Geertman SCM, Van Eck JRR: GIS and models of accessibility potential: an application in planning. *International Journal of Geographical Information Science* 1995, 9:67-80.
16. Khan MM, Ali D, Ferdousy Z, Al-Mamun A: A cost-minimization approach to planning the geographical distribution of health facilities. *Health Policy Plan* 2001, 16:264-272.
17. Crossland MD, Wynne BE, Perkins WC: Spatial decision support systems: An overview of technology and a test of efficacy. *Decision Support Systems* 1995, 14:219-235.
18. Porell FW, Adams EK: Hospital Choice Models: A Review and Assessment of their Utility for Policy Impact Analysis. *Medical Care Research And Review* 1995, 52:158-195.
19. Nyerges T, Jankowski P, Tuthill D, Ramsey K: Collaborative Water Resource Decision Support: Results of a Field Experiment. *Annals of the Association of American Geographers* 2006, 96:699-725.
20. French S: Web-enabled strategic GDSS, e-democracy and Arrow's theorem: A Bayesian perspective. *Decision Support Systems* 2007, 43:1476-1484.
21. Han SH, Yang H, Im D-G: Designing a human-computer interface for a process control room: A case study of a steel manufacturing company. *International Journal of Industrial Ergonomics* 2007, 37:383-393.
22. Hu PJ-H, Ma P-C, Chau PYK: Evaluation of user interface designs for information retrieval systems: a computer-based experiment. *Decision Support Systems* 1999, 27:125-143.
23. Saade RG, Otrakji AC: First impressions last a lifetime: effect of interface type on disorientation and cognitive load. *Computers in Human Behavior* 2007, 23:525-535.
24. Dye AS, Shaw S-L: A GIS-based spatial decision support system for tourists of Great Smoky Mountains National Park. *Journal of Retailing and Consumer Services* 2007, 14:269-278.

25. Bedard Y, Gosselin P, Rivest S, Proulx M-J, Nadeau M, Lebel G, Gag-non M-F: Integrating components with knowledge discovery technology for environmental health decision support. *International Journal of Medical Informatics* 2003, 70:79-94.

26. Jarupathirun S, Zahedi FM: Exploring the influence of perceptual factors in the success of Web-based spatial DSS. *Decision Support Systems* 2007, 43:933-951.

27. Elvins TT, Jain R: Engineering a human factor-based geographic user interface. *Computer Graphics and Applications, IEEE* 1998, 18:66-77.

28. Matthew S, Bambang P: Development of SOVAT: A numerical-spatial decision support system for community health assessment research. *International journal of medical informatics* 2006, 75:771-784.

29. Chen Y-W, Wang C-H, Lin S-J: A multi-objective geographic information system for route selection of nuclear waste transport. *Omega* 2008, 36:363-372.

30. Miranda ML, Galeano MAO, Silva JM, Brown JP, Campbell DS, Coley E, Cowan CS, Harvell D, Lassiter J, Parks JL, Sandelé W: Building Geographic Information System Capacity in Local Health Departments: Lessons From a North Carolina Project. *American Journal of Public Health* 2005, 95:2180-2185.

31. McLafferty S, Grady S: Immigration and Geographic Access to Prenatal Clinics in Brooklyn, NY: A Geographic Information Systems Analysis. *American Journal of Public Health* 2005, 95:638-640.

32. Kamadjeu R, Tolentino H: Web-based public health geographic information systems for resources-constrained environment using scalable vector graphics technology: a proof of concept applied to the expanded program on immunization data. *International Journal of Health Geographics* 2006, 5:24.

33. Deshpande A, Jadad AR: Web 2.0: Could it help move the health system into the 21st century? *The Journal of Men's Health & Gender* 2006, 3:332-336.

34. Barsky E, Purdon M: Introducing Web 2.0: Social networking and social bookmarking for health librarians. *Journal of the Canadian Health Library Associations* 2006, 27:65-67.

35. Greaves M, Mika P: Semantic Web and Web 2.0. *Web Semantics: Science, Services and Agents on the World Wide Web* 2008, 6:1-3.

36. Hendler J, Golbeck J: Metcalfe's law, Web 2.0, and the Semantic Web. *Web Semantics: Science, Services and Agents on the World Wide Web* 2008, 6:14-20.

37. Boulos MNK, Wheeler S: The emerging Web 2.0 social software: an enabling suite of sociable technologies in health and health care education. *Health Information & Libraries Journal* 2007, 24:2-23.

38. Giustini D: Web 3.0 and medicine. *British Medical Journal* 2007, 335:1273-1274.

39. Murugesan S: Understanding Web 2.0. *IT Professional* 2007, 9: 34-41.

40. Cheung K-H, Yip KY, Townsend JP, Scotch M: HCLS 2.0/3.0: Health care and life sciences data mashup using Web 2.0/3.0. *J Biomed Inform* 2008 in press.

41. Bentley R, Appelt W, Busbach U, Hinrichs E, Kerr D, Sikkel K, Trevor J, Woetzel G: Basic support for cooperative work on the World Wide Web. *International Journal of Human-Computer Studies* 1997, 46:827-846.

42. Jones CV: Introduction to the special issue of decision support systems on user interfaces. *Decision Support Systems* 1995, 13:1-2. 43. Bhargava HK, Power DJ, Sun D: Progress in Web-based decision support technologies. *Decision Support Systems* 2007, 43:1083-1095.

44. Currim IS, Gurbaxani V, James, LaBelle, Lim J: Perceptual structure of the desired functionality of Internet-based health information systems. *Health Care Management Science* 2006, 9: 151-170.

45. Jankowski P, Robischon S, Tuthill D, Nyerges T, Ramsey K: Design Considerations and Evaluation of a Collaborative, Spatio-Temporal Decision Support System. *Transactions in GIS* 2006, 10:335-354.

46. Javahery H, Seffah A, Radhakrishnan T: Beyond Power: Making Bioinformatics Tools User-Centered. *Communications of the ACM* 2004, 47:58-63.

47. Bandura A, Locke EA: Negative Self-Efficacy and Goal Effects Revisited. *Journal of Applied Psychology* 2003, 88:87-99.

48. BC Ministries of Health Services and Health Planning: Standards of Accessibility and Guidelines for Provision of Sustainable Acute Care Services by Health Authorities. Victoria: Province of British Columbia; 2002.

49. Moylan JA, Fitzpatrick KT, Beyer AJ, GS G: Factors improving survival in multisystem trauma patients. *Annals of Surgery* 1988, 207:679-685.

50. McGregor J, Hanlon N, Emmons S, Voaklander D, Kelly K: If all ambulances could fly: putting provincial standards of emergency care access to the test in Northern British Columbia. *Canadian journal of rural medicine* 2005, 10:163-168.

51. Boulos MNK: Research protocol: EB-GIS4HEALTH UK –foundation evidence base and ontology-based framework of modular, reusable models for UK/NHS health and healthcare GIS applications. *International Journal of Health Geographics* 2005, 4:2.

52. Kay J: Darwin's marriage and war in Iraq: the missing link. *Financial Times. London* 2008:9.

5

Bridging Rural Health Research and Policy

Dissemination Strategies

Keith J Mueller, Timothy D McBride, Andrew F Coburn, Rebecca T Slifkin, Mary K Wakefield and A Clinton MacKinney

This article describes five strategies that are considered as critical to effective dissemination and expanded use of rural health services research. These include the need for researchers and funders to do the following: engage end users when framing research; tailor the design of products to meet the diverse needs of the end users interested in rural health research; make research products easily accessible to end users; expand contact and working relationships with end users; invest in developing greater capacity for effective dissemination. Besides, the article also discusses the requisite infrastructure to enhance research dissemination. Researchers earn the trust of policy makers when they: present accurate and evidence-based information; acknowledge data or information limitations; provide an objective and nonpartisan viewpoint; work diligently to be recognized experts in their field; respond to user requests in a timely fashion; and provide policy relevant information

Source: Rural Policy Research Institute Health, August, 2007 (www.rupi.org/health).

specific to user needs. Users' need for immediate, relevant, and quality research when the policy is being developed and not after the fact requires that researchers develop an ability to adapt to the needs of users if they want their research to be valued and used.

Introduction

There is widespread agreement that health services research should be more accessible and useful to policy makers and other key stakeholders at the national, state, and local level.[1] This issue has been extensively discussed in the rural health research community for a number of years. In 2000, the conference report, *Linking Rural Health Services Research with Health Policy*,[2] offered detailed recommendations to the research and funding audiences for promoting greater research dissemination and use. More recently, the federal Office of Rural Health Policy has funded the University of North Dakota's Center for Rural Health to strengthen the connection between rural health researchers and important target audiences by identifying the information needs of end users and developing mechanisms for promoting effective research dissemination. Their recent report, *Rural Health Research Gateway: National Audience Needs Study Report*,[3] details the product design and dissemination preferences of key target users of rural health research. In a similar vein, the Rural Policy Research Institute (RUPRI) Health Panel's recent report, *Summary of a Discussion with Congressional Staff on Effective Presentation of Research Results to Policy Stakeholders*,[4] discusses the views of congressional staff users on research dissemination.

Each of these documents identifies a set of issues and potential solutions for expanding policy makers' access to and use of rural health services research through improved products and dissemination. In this paper, the RUPRI Health Panel

1 Throughout this document, the term "users" will be used to refer to legislators, legislative staff, media, advocacy and professional organizations, and other stakeholders.

2 Center for Health Policy Research & Ethics. (2000). *Linking rural health services research with health policy.* Washington, DC: George Mason University Center for Health Policy Research & Ethics. Available at *http://www.gmu.edu/departments/chpre/healthpolicy/briefspublications/GMU_RUPRIrpt.pdf*

3 Moulton, P., Wakefield, M., & Sande, K. (2007). *Rural health research gateway: National audience needs study report.* Grand Forks, ND: University of North Dakota, School of Medicine and Health Sciences, Center for Rural Health. Available at *http://www.nn2.org/docs/Needs_Study_report_020107.pdf*

4 RUPRI Health Panel. (2007). *Summary of a discussion with congressional staff on effective presentation of research results to policy stakeholders.* Columbia, MO: Rural Policy Research Institute.

describes five strategies that these sources and others have identified as critical to effective dissemination and expanded use of rural health services research. These include the need for researchers and funders to do the following:

- Engage end users when framing research.
- Tailor the design of products to meet the diverse needs of the end users interested in rural health research.
- Make research products easily accessible to end users.
- Expand contact and working relationships with end users.
- Invest in developing greater capacity for effective dissemination.

In addition to discussing each of these strategies, this paper discusses the requisite infrastructure needed to enhance research dissemination.

Key Strategies

Engage End Users when Framing Research

Rural researchers should anticipate users' needs by developing long-term agendas that consider emerging rural health issues. One of the common complaints made by users is that the research they need is rarely readily available. Rural researchers should engage users in framing their research agendas. Strategies might include:

- Establish a "research to policy network" comprised researchers and users. Such a network could both help the research community understand and anticipate users' information needs and assist users in gaining familiarity with the broad knowledge base available through the research community.
- Develop additional "synthesis" products that summarize in an accessible, readable format what is currently known on a topic to identify needed additional research.

The process of conceiving and executing a research study often requires substantially more time than the timeframes typically followed by policy makers. However, while it may not always be possible to anticipate specific policy issues that will be relevant in the near future, by structuring research around broader themes that have been identified by policy makers as of interest, the chances of researchers possessing both the expertise and the data needed to answer more focused questions as they arise are improved. Researchers and others should monitor policy developments so that previously released research findings are communicated when they are relevant to current policy debates.

Tailor the Design of Products to Meet the Diverse Needs of the End Users Interested in Rural Health Research

It is important to recognize that different products are needed for different stakeholder groups. Thus, research delivered to policy audiences must be packaged to fit the needs of and appeal to the audience. Policy makers prefer short, to-the-point, user-friendly products, such as policy briefs or summary fact sheets that contain key information relevant to policy discussions. Policy briefs containing key descriptive findings can be disseminated while the researcher is preparing a journal article. Peer-reviewed journal articles often do not meet the needs of users who seek timely research translated into accessible language. However, journal articles remain important to users as an additional source of information that reinforces the credibility of the research. Some users report regularly perusing certain journals, specifically *Health Affairs*, *The New England Journal of Medicine,* and *The Journal of the American Medical Association.*

Policy briefs or other dissemination products should have well-written titles that reflect key "takeaways" from the research and that grab the attention of the user to read further. Products should include strategic visuals (such as simple and clear graphs/charts) and colors, but should avoid superfluous pictures. Detailed information on local areas (e.g., states, counties, congressional districts) appeals to policy makers, since "all politics is local" even if the issue is national. The products should be structured to include key findings easily found by the reader, contact information for the authors (including internet links if available), policy or practice implications, references, and sources for further information. Users emphasize that every research product must include policy recommendations in the context of legislative realities. Users need to know the limitations of the analysis, but information about the methods, beyond sample size and the date data collected, should be available as references or through internet links.

Make Research Products Easily Accessible to End Users

Research utilization is predicated on users having ready access to research findings. Users need research results in seconds or minutes, not hours or days.

Multiple communication channels are needed to reach various audiences, including policy makers, associations, advocacy groups, and media. Users indicate that traditional communication vehicles for research findings, including conference presentations and peer-reviewed publications, are not a primary information source; they report that electronic and verbal communications are preferred delivery modes.

Users prefer e-mail announcements with links to new research findings. This allows for timely access to information and actively routes documents directly to interested parties. In addition, well-designed and easy-to-use websites direct users to relevant research findings. A single electronic portal to facilitate easy access to relevant rural research findings was cited as an important information source, rather than relying on finding multiple websites. Websites should be professionally designed, have search capabilities, connect to all other rural research centers, and be tested for ease of usability and usefulness to ensure that barriers to accessing information are eliminated. Virtually all research products produced in paper form should be electronically available.

Expand Contact and Working Relationships with End Users

Perhaps the most effective means of disseminating research to policy users is through direct, interpersonal contact. For rural health research to inform policy, users must trust that the information they receive is reliable and credible. They will often rely on personal contacts with researchers they trust. Sustained and substantive communication engenders trust. Specific users of policy research change frequently, so researchers must regularly renew efforts to establish and nurture relationships. Obvious points of contact for researchers include locally based users and policy makers with jurisdictional responsibility in the topic area of the research. Occasionally, special relationships may be built because a policy research user becomes familiar with the researcher's work and as a result trusts the judgment of that researcher.

Researchers need not be the primary contact for policy users in order to communicate research findings at critical times. Intermediaries can connect the researcher's work to policy activity. The most typical example would be advocacy groups using research findings, with the credibility of the work resting with the researcher but the timely input being the role of the group. Researchers can take advantage of this conduit by providing unambiguous results (not subject to interpretation) to the groups.

Researchers earn the trust of policy makers when they:

- Present accurate and evidence-based information.
- Acknowledge data or information limitations.
- Provide an objective and nonpartisan viewpoint.
- Work diligently to be recognized experts in their field.
- Respond to user requests in a timely fashion.
- Provide policy relevant information specific to user needs.

Researchers should provide timely and objective analysis, even if it may conflict with established policy views. Although researcher-policy maker relationships develop best through interpersonal interaction, trust also can develop through electronic communication or shared written documents.

Invest in Developing Greater Capacity for Effective Dissemination

Effective dissemination efforts require dedicated resources to support specialized communication skills, in addition to the resources needed for the research activity. Policy communication skills are particularly important for the development and dissemination of products valuable to policy audiences, e.g., writing effective press releases alerting potential users to new research output. Thus, new skills may be needed to complement those of research teams.

The imperative to produce timely, useful, and accessible information creates a competitive pressure for many researchers; i.e., should researchers dedicate limited resources (time, dollars, and people) to produce material for users or to produce scholarly publications? Managing this conflict is possible with a combination of the following:

- Dedicate resources and staff time to dissemination; e.g., fund staff positions designated for information dissemination and provide media skills and/or writing training to certain researchers.
- Include specific funding requests for information dissemination to users during grant application or cooperative agreement processes.
- Recognize that if funding is limited there will be a tradeoff between the quantity of research and dedicating resources to dissemination. Negotiate the allocation of resources with the funding agency.
- Consider all available resources for dissemination, including public relations units within universities, the Rural Assistance Center, associations, and dissemination units within funding agencies.

Researchers should have a business plan and budget for effective dissemination that identifies resources consistent with a menu of options to meet the needs of policy makers, trade organization, and practitioners, including:

- Writers, e.g., science writer, journalist,
- Public relations, and
- Publications budget, including website development and management, support for telephonic and electronic communications, travel to sustain relationships, and staff time for dissemination.

Critical to all of the considerations regarding resources for dissemination is recognition by the funding source that dedicated resources are required for effective dissemination. The same tradeoffs that confront researchers confront funding agencies. If expectations are imposed on researchers to be more effective in dissemination and there are no new resources provided, funding agencies will need to adjust expectations for the volume of research activity.

Implications

This paper outlines strategies to enhance the use of rural health research by users through more effective dissemination. Evidence from focus groups conducted by the University of North Dakota for the Federal Office of Rural Health Policy and other sources indicates several broad strategies, described above, for improving the effectiveness of dissemination. The analysis presented here has several implications for the efforts of researchers, for their institutions, and for agencies granting funds for policy-related health services research.

Implications for Research Project Development

Researchers need to be proactive in thinking about the applications of their rural health policy work to the development of health policies, beginning in the project development phase and continuing all the way through the completion of final reports. Researchers need to identify and seek resources to help them fund dissemination efforts throughout the project, but especially as project results are obtained and can be disseminated.

Implications for Timely Dissemination

Researchers should consider users' needs when developing research project timelines and dissemination strategies. Users' need for immediate, relevant, and quality research when the policy is being developed and not after the fact requires that researchers develop an ability to adapt to the needs of users if they want their research to be valued and used. Researchers also need to be responsive to requests for data and analysis in a timely fashion, even if the research results are final but not yet in published form. This requires developing relationships with users and nurturing those relationships. In addition, researchers need to develop and enhance their skills in the areas of research dissemination. Finally, researchers should develop the ability to use multiple methods to deliver research findings in a timely fashion, including the media, who are an effective intermediary between researchers, the public, and users.

Implications for Program Announcements

Federal granting agencies need to be proactive to encourage researchers to develop dissemination strategies throughout their projects. This includes not only providing the carrots of funds and resources to help researchers develop the infrastructure to disseminate research at their home institution and through a central location such as the Rural Health Research Gateway, but also the stick to require that all policy-relevant health services research have a dissemination plan to policy and/or practice.

(Keith J Mueller, Ph.D., is a Professor and the Director of the RUPRI Center for Rural Health Policy Analysis at the University of Nebraska Medical Center. He was the 1996-7 President of the National Rural Health Association and the recipient of the Association's Distinguished Rural Health Researcher Award in 1998. He served a four-year term on the National Advisory Committee on Rural Health and Human Services, and serves on the Advisory Panel on Medicare Education for the Centers for Medicare and Medicaid Services. He has published more than 40 articles on health planning, access to care for vulnerable populations, rural health, and access to care among the uninsured. Dr. Mueller has directed major health services studies funded by the US Agency for Healthcare Research and Quality, the Federal Office of Rural Health Policy, and the Robert Wood Johnson Foundation. He has testified on numerous occasions before committees of Congress and in other forums, including the Institute of Medicine and the Medicare Payment Advisory Commission.

Timothy D McBride, Ph.D., is a Professor of Health Management and Policy in the School of Public Health at St. Louis University. Dr. McBride's research focuses on public economics, with special emphasis on the economics of aging and health. In the health policy area, Dr. McBride's research has focused on Medicare policy reform, the uninsured, long-term care, rural health, and healthcare reform. He is the author of over 25 research articles, book chapters, and monographs. Dr. McBride joined St. Louis University in 2003 after spending 13 years at University of Missouri-St. Louis and four years at the Urban Institute in Washington, DC.

Andrew F Coburn, Ph.D., is a Professor of Health Policy and Management and directs the Institute for Health Policy in the Muskie School of Public Service at the University of Southern Maine. Dr. Coburn is a senior investigator in the Maine Rural Health Research Center and has published extensively on rural health issues related to health insurance coverage and long-term care. He is a contributing author of the book Rural Health in the United States published in 1999 by the Oxford University Press.

Rebecca T Slifkin, Ph.D., is the Director of the North Carolina Rural Health Research and Policy Analysis Center, one of eight centers funded by the federal Office of Rural Health Policy. She is also Director of the Program on Healthcare Economics and Finance at the Cecil G. Sheps Center for Health Services Research at the University of North Carolina at Chapel Hill, and a Research Associate Professor in the Department of Social Medicine in the Medical School. Her work has spanned a broad array of topics, including Medicare payments, Medicaid managed care, Critical Access Hospitals, and access to care for rural minorities.

Mary K Wakefield, Ph.D., R.N., is Professor and Director of the Center for Rural Health at the University of North Dakota. Before assuming her current responsibilities, Dr. Wakefield was Professor and Director of the Center for Health Policy at George Mason University, Fairfax, Virginia. From January 1993 to January 1996, Dr. Wakefield was the Chief of Staff for United States Senator Kent Conrad (D-ND). Prior to that she served as Legislative Assistant and Chief of Staff to Senator Quentin Burdick (D-ND). Throughout her tenure on Capitol Hill, Dr. Wakefield advised on a range of public health policy issues, drafted legislative proposals, and worked with interest groups and other Senate offices. From 1987 to 1992, she co-chaired the Senate Rural Health Caucus Staff Organization. Dr. Wakefield served on President Clinton's Advisory Commission on Consumer Protection and Quality in the Healthcare Industry. She was appointed to the Institute of Medicine's Committee on Quality of Healthcare in America and is a member of the Medicare Payment Advisory Commission.

A Clinton MacKinney, M.D., M.S., is a board-certified family physician delivering emergency medicine services in rural Minnesota. Dr. MacKinney also works as a senior consultant for Stroudwater Associates, a rural hospital consulting firm. Lastly, Dr. MacKinney is a contract researcher for the RUPRI Center for Rural Health Policy Analysis at the University of Nebraska Medical Center. Prior to these positions, Dr. MacKinney served as the medical director for a large primary care practice and practiced full-time family medicine for 14 years in rural Iowa. Dr. MacKinney graduated from the Medical College of Ohio in 1982 and completed a family practice residency through the Mayo healthcare system in 1985. He maintains family practice board certification and a Geriatric Certificate of Added Qualifications. In 1998, Dr. MacKinney completed his master's degree in administrative medicine from the University of Wisconsin. Dr. MacKinney's professional interests include healthcare quality improvement, organizational performance improvement, physician-administration relationships, rural health policy, and population-based medicine.)

Section II

Practices

6

National Centre of Rural Medicine in Norway
A Bridge from Rural Practice to the Academy

IJ Aaraas and E Swensen

Context: ***Rural medical practice in Norway has an honourable 400 year history, but this has diminished since the end of World War II. Despite official intention to support a decentralised population, rural and remote populations have continuously reduced in Norway over the last 10 years. A consequence of the accompanying reduction in rural and remote GP services has been a distinct reduction in opportunities for medical students and intern placements. In 1999 the University of Tromso implemented some projects to stimulate rural medical practice, funded by the government. This culminated in the 2007 foundation of the Norwegian National Centre of Rural Medicine (NCRM) in Tromso.***

Issue: A key challenge of the NCRM is to identify factors that influence young doctors to choose rural careers. This is reflected in the three concurrent aims or perspectives of the NCRM: (1) to bridge the gap between the academy and rural medical practice (the principal perspective); (2) to promote research, education and networking among rural health professionals (the operational perspective); and

Source: Rural and Remote Health Issue 1, Volume 8, January-March 2008 (www.rrh.org.au).

(3) to contribute to the recruitment, stability and quality of rural healthcare (the political perspective).

Lessons learned: The NCRM has had a number of achievements that include a publication that provides a narrative perspective on rural practice, the role of the rural doctor, and how rural culture and context influence proper clinical decision-making. Another achievement is a professional development and research program that has been successful in fostering a number of major studies, and led to the formation of a supportive PhD research group. The NCRM has also facilitated networking between rural practitioners and academics, at conferences and via its rural doctor website, and promoted cooperative international activities. In these ways the NCRM has fostered the transformation of rural doctors' experience into theory to enhance medical knowledge, begun to redress the balance between community- and hospital-based services, and so made a favourable start to building a bridge between rural practice and the medical academy in Norway.

Context

Honourable History

In Norway, rural public health doctors have a long and honourable history dating back to 1603 when the first doctor was employed by the state as a regional medical officer in Western Norway. Government employment of rural doctors then continued for almost 400 years until 1984. During the twentieth century, and particularly after World War II, hospital specialists have gradually overtaken the leadership and influence of their rural colleagues. The *Municipality Health Act 1984* compounded this when it determined that the main employer of rural doctors should be the municipality, rather than the state.

Centralisation and Rural Deprivation

In Norway, as in other western countries, the trend in the health service system has been towards urbanization and rural deprivation. Since 2000 the Norwegian transformation of specialist healthcare, including hospitals, into state enterprises has contributed to increasing centralization of the medical workforce, at the expense of services to rural and remote areas. This has happened despite Norway's inclusion in the group of European countries with an agreement to support a decentralised population. Although the Norwegian Government has supported certain initiatives (e.g., tutorial groups for residents) to stimulate recruitment and retention of rural and remote health workers, the challenges described by WONCA[1] before 2000 remain:

> *The world wide shortage of rural family doctors contributes directly to the difficulties with providing adequate medical care in rural areas in both developed and less developed countries. WONCA believes that there is an urgent need to implement strategies to educate, recruit and support sufficient numbers of skilled rural family doctors to provide the necessary services.*

In all rural and remote Norwegian municipalities there has been population reduction in each of the last 10 years[2]. During the same period there has been an increasing instability among GPs in small and remote municipalities[3], resulting in a distinct reduction in opportunities for medical student and intern placements. At the University of Tromso, where the rural placement of medical students has been a core element of the curriculum since the founding of the medical school in 1973[4], this unprecedented situation is impacting on the quality of medical education.

Foundation of an Academic Centre for Rural Medicine

In 1999 the University of Tromsø's proposed project strategies to stimulate teaching, research and networking among rural practitioners were approved and financed by the Ministry of Health. Initially based in the north, the projects have developed into nationwide activity, culminating in the designation of the National Centre of Rural Medicine (NCRM) in Tromsø as the permanent Norwegian academic centre for rural practice from 2007 (Figures 1, 2). Today the centre is funded and professionally supported by three partners: the Norwegian Directorate of Social and Health Affairs; Health North (the state corporation for specialist health services in the northern region); and the University of Tromsø. The funding of the NCRM acknowledges the failure of economic incentives and government campaigns to motivate young doctors to choose a rural career, even under optimal economic and political conditions.

Figure 1: Map Showing the Location of Norway in Northern Europe

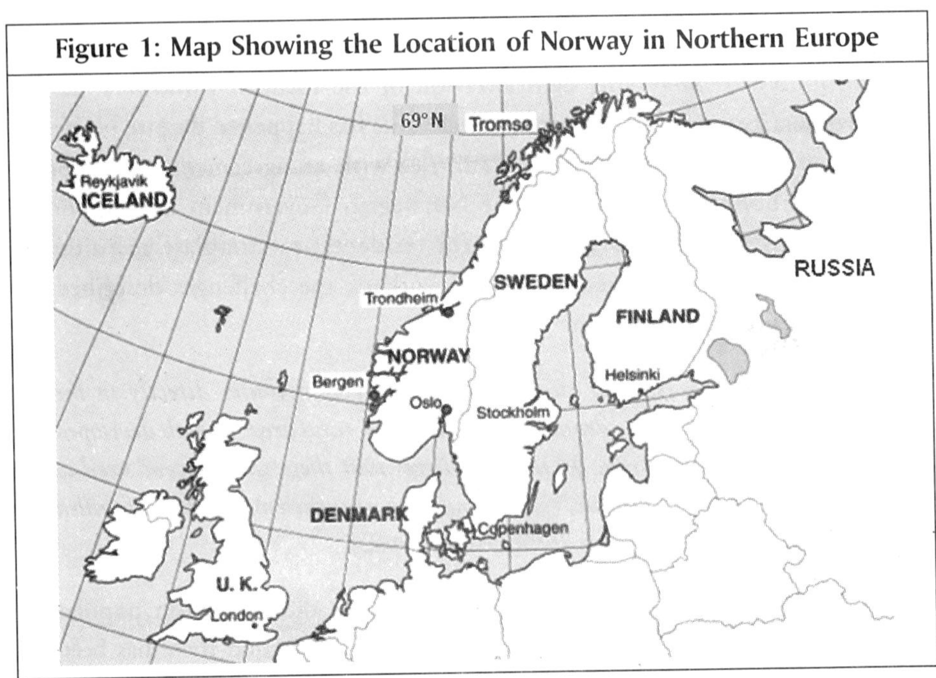

Figure 2: Tromsø – The Home of the National Centre of Rural Medicine in Norway

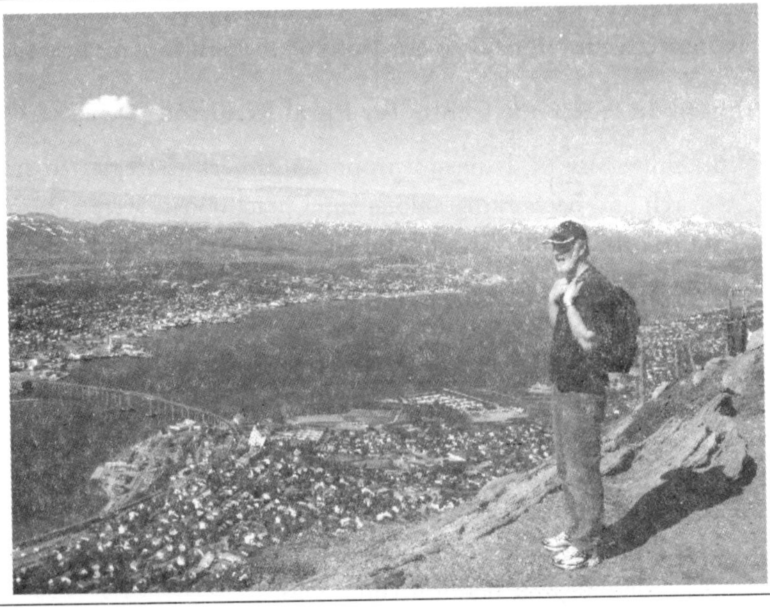

Issue

The NCRM was dedicated to examining both common and diverse expressions and values of rural practice, and to use this insight and knowledge to revitalise and strengthen the healthcare provided to rural-living populations. A key challenge for the NCRM is to identify factors that influence young doctors to choose rural careers. This article presents and discusses the NCRM's main aims and achievements to date.

Aims

The NCRM has three main aims. The first and *principal* aim is to bridge the gap between the academy and rural medical practice. The second *operational* aim is to promote research, education and networking among rural health professionals. The third *political* aim is to contribute to recruitment, stability and quality in rural healthcare.

The principal aim implies that rural medical *practice* what is expected from the rural family doctor and how he/she actually delivers it needs to be investigated, described and interpreted. Bridging the gap between practice and the academy specifically means integrating the rural perspective into medical *theory* and the body of medical *knowledge*. The operational aim is the core activity, fundamental to the academic centre, thereby contributing to the other two aims. The NCRM's political aim depends on coordinated work to promote empirical and research-based evidence aimed at improving rural practice and healthcare, and influencing relevant bodies to provide appropriate resources.

Achievements

Among a variety of activities and achievements, three will be discussed. The first is a book, which has encouraged a national collegial discussion about the concept and nature of rural medicine. The second is a professional development and research program that has consolidated the basis from which to continue the NCRM. The third is an innovation of networking and meeting places for rural doctors primarily national but also international aimed at enhancing opportunities to share experience, build theory and discuss professional development issues.

Published descriptions and distinctions of rural medicine: This 2005 Norwegian language book (English title: Between nostalgia and avant-garde – rural medicine in modern times) consists of 13 essays[5]. Among these, five concern historical and theoretical perspectives of rural medicine, and the remaining eight are based on rural GPs experiences and stories from their own practice. The book created considerable discussion among the Norwegian medical establishment. The editors declared intention was to be open to various interpretations of rural medicine, rather than narrowing the concept of rural medicine to any particular tradition. Among the criticism, one academic criticised the book as being imbalanced to the point of nostalgia and ideology, and so inappropriately addressing today's rural health challenges[6].

In 2007 the NCRM arranged a workshop with international narrative medicine scholar Professor Rita Charon[7] at Columbia University, New York, to explore rural medicine perspectives. In support of the NCRM publication, the workshop endorsed the common experience in the stories of illness shared by this expert and rural practitioners, and the fundamental value of narrative as providing examples of good clinical performance. In rural practice, narratives related to illness, family, culture, context and life history often contain information crucial to appropriate patient-centred understanding and decision-making. This corresponds to the common features of rural living, which are highly relevant to the rural doctor. Based on lifelong experience as a rural GP, and in accordance with the diverse perspectives of the NCRM book, one of the authors of this article [ES] has identified some comparative dimensions that describe key differences between urban and rural determinants and values (Figure 3). Subsequent workshop and educational discussions in a variety of settings suggest these differences are consistent with the general views of doctors and medical students in Norway and other European countries.

Professional development and research: The NCRM *Program for professional development and research* was one of the initial joint projects of the University of Tromsø and the Ministry of Health. Launched in 1999, its aim was to stimulate quality improvement and research among rural GPs. Since its inception, the program has supported approximately 50 minor projects run by GPs, either alone

Figure 3: Summary of Key Differences between Urban and Rural Determinants and Values

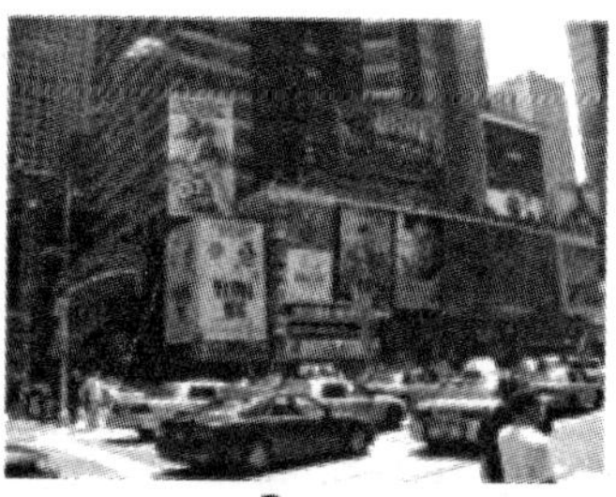

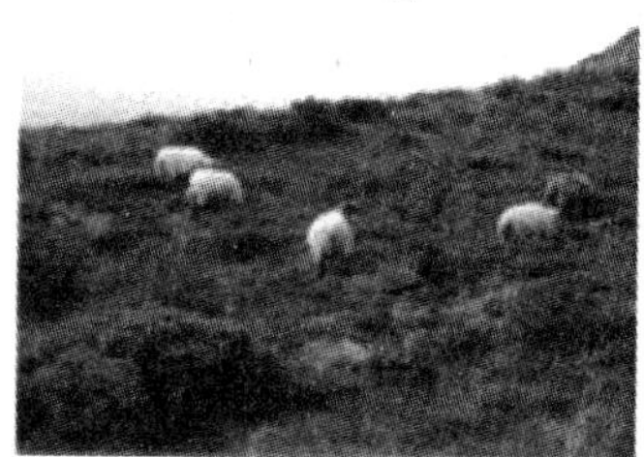

Urban	Rural
• Infrastructure	• Weather
• Friends	• Family
• Consuming	• Land
• Individuality	• Community
• Documents	• Stories

or with other local health professionals. Among these, seven projects have expanded into major PhD research, constituting a varied portfolio of themes:

1. A hermeneutical approach to understanding rural practice.
2. Communication and understanding the risks of medical decision-making.
3. The workload, work content, and the interaction of public health physicians in Norway.
4. Medical leadership in rural practice.
5. The role and tasks of the doctor in emergency teamwork.
6. Care of people suffering from dementia in northern rural practices.
7. The use of hospital specialist services from different municipalities.

Based on this, the NCRM has established a PhD research group among rural GPs. The group meets on a regular basis for mutual guidance and feedback, with participants granted part-time appointments to the centre to enhance their ability to combine research with clinical work.

Research strategy: In the beginning, NCRM research strategy was simply to support and motivate individual initiatives among GPs; however, two main thematic areas are on the future agenda. The first is to investigate and describe aspects of rural practice; and the second, to explore the specific challenges of and possibilities for shared care between rural-based practitioners and hospital-based specialists. We believe the latter concern to be of particular importance in Norway where primary healthcare and hospital care function as separate enterprises, both economically and professionally. The rising hospital costs of many years have now reached enormous heights and are practically out of control. The logical solution is to promote shared care and allocate more resources (money, manpower, education and research) to developing primary and rural healthcare[8].

Networking: The third main achievement of NCRM is creation of meeting places for and networking among rural practitioners and academics. Over the years the centre has promoted this by arranging annual national conferences on rural medicine, along with offering a virtual rural doctor meeting space on the website. The NCRM has also brought the Norwegian discussion to an international agenda on several occasions by its participation in the European Rural and Isolated Practitioners Association (EURIPA) and in two workshops on defining and describing rural medicine (WONCA World Rural Conference, Santiago de Compostela, 2003; and WONCA Europe Conference, Paris, 2007). Other international initiatives include involvement in a student rural placement exchange, and contribution to an internationally renowned film on doctor-patient communication in a rural community[9].

Nationally, the networking activities have been essential to NCRM achievements to date, and the future intention is to serve as a home base, a meeting place and an arena for development and debate. Internationally, the NCRM has been restrained by a language barrier, for few Norwegian patients, especially those who are elderly, speak English and this limits participation in the exchange of students among rural practices. In addition the NCRM website is still under development and does not yet have an English version. However, in the meantime, many Norwegian students and doctors are fluent in English, and are interested and involved in international networking activities.

Conclusion

The existence of a rural medical academy is crucial for long-term recruitment to and retention of the rural medical workforce, and also to maintain a balance between community- and hospital-based services. It is also important to convert rural doctors experience into theory for the further development of medical knowledge and healthcare. Considering its achievements to date, the NCRM has made a favourable start to building a bridge between rural practice and the medical academy in Norway.

(IJ Aaraas and E Swensen, National Centre of Rural Medicine, University of Tromsø, Kommunlegekontoret, Norway).

References

1. WONCA. *Rural practice and rural health.* (Online) 1999. Available: *http://www.globalfamily doctor.com/aboutWonca/ working_groups/rural_training/practice/Practi_t.htm* (Accessed 5 June 2008).
2. Statistisk sentralbyrå [Statistics Norway]. *Fortsatt sentralisering* [Continuing centralization]. (Online) 2007. Available: *http://www. ssb.no/vis/emner/00/01/20/valgaktuelt/art-2007-08-30-01.html* (Accessed 30 August 2007). [In Norwegian]
3. Andersen F, Forsdahl A, Herder O, Aaraas IJ. Legemangelen I distriktene nordnorske funn, nasjonale utfordringer [Lack of doctors in rural districts the situation in Northern Norway]. *Tidsskr Nor Legeforen* 2001; 121: 2732-2735. (In Norwegian)
4. Knutsen SF, Johnsen R, Forsdahl A. Practical training of medical students in community medicine. Eight years experience from the University of Tromsø. *Scandinavian Journal of Primary Healthcare* 1986; 4: 109-114.
5. Lian OS, Merok E (Eds). *Mellom nostalgi og avantgarde. Distriktsmedisinen i moderne tid.* Kristiansand: Høyskoleforlaget, 2005. (In Norwegian)
6. Hunskår S. Fri oss fra den nye distriktsmedisinen. [Free us from the new rural medicine!] *Tidsskr Nor Legeforen* 2005; 125: 1879. (In Norwegian)
7. Charon R. *Narrative medicine. Honouring the stories of illness.* Oxford: Oxford University Press, 2006.
8. Macinko J, Starfield B, Shi L. The contribution of primary care systems to health outcomes within Organization for Economic Cooperation and Development (OECD) countries, 1970-1998. *Health Services Research* 2003; 38(3): 831-865.
9. Swensen E. Et hermeneutisk ballespark [Interview with Eivind Gustav Olsen Merok]. *Tidsskr Nor Legeforen* 2005; 125: 3304-3305. (In Norwegian).

Quality through Collaboration

The Future of Rural & Frontier Emergency Medical Services in the US Health System

This article initially discusses how improving the quality of healthcare services has become a key focus of the healthcare industry, State and Federal government payers, commercial insurers, employers, and increasingly, patients and the general public in the context of the US. Subsequently, a five-pronged strategy to address the quality challenges in rural communities. The first strategy is to adopt an integrated, priority approach to addressing both personal and population health needs at the community level. The second strategy is to establish a stronger quality improvement support structure to rural health systems and professionals in acquiring knowledge and tools to improve quality. The next is to enhance the human resource capacity of rural communities, including the education, training, and deployment of healthcare professionals, and the preparedness of rural residents to engage actively in improving their health and healthcare. The fourth is to monitor rural healthcare systems to ensure that they are financially stable and provide assistance in securing the necessary capital for system

---

Source: www.hrsa.gov. Reprinted with permission.

redesign. The last strategy is to invest in building Information and Communication Technology (ICT) infrastructure, which has enormous potential to enhance health and healthcare over the coming decade.

Integrating Rural EMS into the Healthcare Quality Debate

Improving the quality of healthcare services has become a key focus of the healthcare industry, State and Federal government payors, commercial insurers, employers, and increasingly, patients and the general public. Federal agencies such as the Centers for Medicare and Medicaid Services (CMS) are exploring ways to reimburse healthcare providers for delivering effective, high quality services (a strategy usually referred to as "pay for performance.") Employer coalitions such as the Leapfrog Group are looking for ways to reduce medical errors, encourage public reporting of clinical outcomes, and reward doctors and hospitals for improving quality and safety. Provider coalitions such as the Hospital Quality Alliance (HQA), a joint effort of the American Hospital Association, the Federation of American Hospitals, and the Association of American Medical Colleges (along with CMS and the Joint Commission on the Accreditation of Healthcare Organizations), are urging hospitals to permit an array of clinical quality measures to be reported publicly on the CMS-run Hospital Compare website (*www.hospitalcompare.hhs.gov*).

What about Rural?

Unfortunately, rural healthcare has been only peripherally involved in these discussions. Rural healthcare leaders and advocates, however, are keenly interested in integrating rural issues into the quality debate. With the November 2004 publication of *Quality through Collaboration: The Future of Rural Health*, the Institute of Medicine's Committee on the Future of Rural Healthcare charted an agenda for rural communities to fulfill the six aims set forth in the Institute of Medicine's 2001 report *Crossing the Quality Chasm: A New Health System for the 21st Century* to make healthcare safe, effective, patient-centered, timely, efficient, and equitable. The Institute of Medicine (IOM) committee on the Future of

Rural Healthcare proposed a five-pronged strategy to address the quality challenges in rural communities:

Strategy 1: Adopt an integrated, priority approach to addressing both personal and population health needs at the community level.

Strategy 2: Establish a stronger quality improvement support structure to rural health systems and professionals in acquiring knowledge and tools to improve quality.

Strategy 3: Enhance the human resource capacity of rural communities, including the education, training, and deployment of healthcare professionals, and the preparedness of rural residents to engage actively in improving their health and healthcare.

Strategy 4: Monitor rural healthcare systems to ensure that they are financially stable and provide assistance in securing the necessary capital for system redesign.

Strategy 5: Invest in building an Information and Communication Technology (ICT) infrastructure, which has enormous potential to enhance health and healthcare over the coming decade.

The Institute of Medicine believes that adoption and implementation of this multi-faceted strategy is necessary to enhance quality, to build focused rural community health *systems*, and to bring rural providers fully into the national debate on improving healthcare quality, safety, and performance.

So where does EMS fit in the "Quality Agenda?"

In its 2004 report, the Committee on the Future of Rural Health explicitly recognized EMS as part of the *core set* of healthcare services that are of greatest need in rural areas, while also noting concerns regarding insufficient access to EMS because of constraints caused by long-standing shortages of qualified EMS professionals in many rural areas. They also recognized the importance of EMS in ensuring timely care in emergency situations, and the unique aspects of rural EMS due to long distances to definitive care. The committee further noted that because rural care processes are different from those in urban areas, the data that are necessary for quality improvement purposes are different. They pointed out that data on emergency care, stabilization and transfer services are of great importance in rural areas, and EMS involvement in quality improvement efforts is, therefore, critical.

This paper was created with the purpose of serving as a companion document to *Quality Through Collaboration*. The focus is to encourage policy makers, healthcare providers, and most importantly, EMS officials and providers, to recognize the importance of including rural and frontier EMS in the national discussion about healthcare quality. It is meant to promote discussion regarding specific ways that rural and frontier Emergency Medical Services (EMS) providers can engage in the rural healthcare quality movement.

Specifically, the objectives of the paper are to:

1) Provide recommendations on building the best possible emergency care "system" in rural America. These recommendations will be presented in a framework based on the five strategies outlined in *Quality Through Collaboration*, but other recent studies and reports will also be examined in detail. Improving the quality of emergency care has been an important (and in some cases primary) focus of other influential publications in recent years including the *Rural Hospital Flexibility Program Strategic Plan*, the *Rural and Frontier EMS Agenda for the Future, The HRSA Model Trauma System Planning and Evaluation* and the IOM *Future of Emergency Care* series (which includes *Hospital-Based Emergency Care: at the Breaking Point*, *Emergency Medical Services at the Crossroads*, and *Emergency Care for Children: Growing Pains*).

2) Propose new opportunities for collaboration to further rural EMS quality of care among key stakeholders in rural EMS including the National Association of State EMS Officials; the National Organization of State Offices of Rural Health, the National Rural Health Association and other rural health advocates; EMS collaboratives such as the North Central EMS Institute, Critical Illness and Trauma Foundation, rural health resource and technical assistance centers including the Rural Emergency Medical Services and Trauma Technical Assistance Center, Federally-funded rural health research centers, and Federal agencies including the Office of Rural Health Policy, NTHSA, CMS and others.

Organization of this Document

The five priority strategies in *Quality Through Collaboration* will be addressed in turn. In each section, following a discussion of the IOM rural quality report, recommendations from other key policy reports that related to the IOM recommendations will be listed. Each bullet is followed by parentheses to show the source of the recommendation (FSP = *FLEX Program Strategic Plan*, RFEMS = *Rural and Frontier EMS Agenda for the Future*; MTSPE = *Model Trauma System Planning and Evaluation*, IOM-FEC = IOM *Future of Emergency Care* series). A brief description of each of these documents is presented in Appendix A.

Particular attention will be given to key themes that are shared in common among the reports mentioned above. By bringing attention to key consistent themes in these recent reports, the authors hope to create an active dialogue across the traditional "silos" of rural health and Emergency Medical Services, which could lead to the development of a well-funded, broad-based model rural EMS system that would help ensure access to high quality emergency care in America's rural and frontier areas.

Quality through Collaboration: Priority Strategies

Strategy I: An Integrated Approach to Improving Health

The first strategy proposed by the IOM Committee on the Future of Rural Health was to formulate an integrated approach to addressing the personal healthcare and population health needs of rural communities. The report provides a broad range of actions that could be adopted at both the personal healthcare system level and the community level to improve health status. They suggested an integrated framework that would lead to a more optimal allocation of scarce financial resources devoted to improving the quality of health in rural communities.

One specific point of discussion in *Quality Through Collaboration* in this discussion related to EMS was:

> *Timely access to emergency care is a primary concern for rural citizens. The IOM committee recognizes timely care as something different in rural and urban areas, and in rural communities', emergency care is the primary concern in regard to timely care.*

The report points out that residents who are far from a source of definitive care depend on EMS to ensure that they receive timely access to care. This means EMS must: 1) be adequately equipped to care for patients who may have long travel distances before reaching a hospital; 2) be able to communicate with Emergency Department (ED) physicians and specialists to ensure appropriate, timely medical direction, and 3) be able to transport patients as quickly and as safely as possible. The key role EMS plays in ensuring timely access to care also is reflected in numerous recommendations of the *Flex Program Strategic Plan*, *Rural and Frontier EMS Agenda for the Future*, the *Model Trauma System Planning and Evaluation*, and the *Future of Emergency Care* series.

These recommendations include:

- Promote integration of rural EMS operations into local networks and other activities designed to strengthen rural EMS. [FSP].
- Plan, integrate and regulate, at the State level, aero-medical, critical care transport, and other state-wide or region-wide systems of specialty care and transportation. Consider the evolving role of telehealth resources and their application to EMS patient management and medical oversight .... [RFEMS, Clinical Care & Transportation Decisions/Resources Chapter].
- Facilitate a State-level process, guided by an appropriate multi-disciplinary committee, to ensure inclusive systems of trauma care and other time critical emergency care that define the roles of rural and frontier hospitals.... [RFEMS, Clinical Care & Transportation Decisions/Resources Chapter].
- The emergency care system of the future should be one in which all participants (from 9-1-1 to ambulances to EDs) fully coordinate their activities and integrate communications to ensure seamless emergency.
- The Federal government should support the development of national standards for emergency care performance measurement; categorization of all emergency care facilities; and protocols for the treatment, triage, and transport of prehospital patients [IOM-FEC].

In addition, the IOM *Quality Through Collaboration* report notes the high death rate of unintentional injury in rural areas, an issue of specific interest to EMS:

There are salient differences between rural and urban communities in terms of health behaviors and environmental threats that must be addressed to improve community health. One threat to health highlighted in the IOM report is the age-adjusted death rate for unintentional injury that is much higher in both males and females in rural areas than in urban environments.

Addressing the issue of unintentional injury is a natural fit for rural EMS providers. EMS is a critical part of the trauma system that addresses the continuum of care: from prevention to treatment to rehabilitation for unintentional injuries. In rural areas, reducing rates of unintentional injuries will have a marked impact on community health status. Reducing rates of unintentional injury is one of the key objectives derived from *Healthy People 2010*, a document based on a broad consultation process, built on the best scientific knowledge, and designed to measure programs over time. Unintentional injury is one of ten leading health indicators in *Healthy People 2010*, and the leading causes of unintentional injury, motor vehicle crashes and homicides, are often predictable and preventable. By becoming engaged in prevention of unintentional injury, rural EMS can have a considerable impact on local communities.

Related recommendations *from other policy documents include:*

- Make prevention one of the EMS-based community health service roles of adequately staffed rural/frontier EMS provider agencies [RFEMSA, Prevention Chapter].
- Among local, State, Federal, and national EMS and public health agencies (and other agencies with prevention roles), cooperatively develop and fund community health advocacy roles and prevention programs for rural/frontier EMS personnel that are mutually beneficial [RFEMSA, Prevention Chapter].
- Federal agencies and national organizations with prevention roles should channel existing [injury prevention] programs through State EMS agencies to local EMS provider agencies [RFEMSA, Prevention Chapter].
- Provider agency policy/procedures and innovative incentives, EMS curricula, and accreditation, and other standards target EMS provider health, safety and prevention [RFEMSA, Prevention Chapter].

- The trauma system should contribute to reducing the entire burden of injury in a State, region, or community. Therefore, it should integrate all three phases of injury prevention into planning and practice. The trauma system should produce improved health status outcomes, such as reduced injury occurrence and better clinical outcomes for injured patients [MTSPE, Three Phases of Injury Prevention Chapter].
- Emergency care is broader than EMS and encompasses the full continuum of services involved in emergency medical care, including EMS, hospital-based ED and trauma care, specialty care, bystander care, and injury prevention [IOM – FEC EMS: *At the Crossroads*].

Strategy II: Quality Improvement Activities in Rural Areas

Chapter Two of *Quality Through Collaboration* emphasizes the unique needs of rural healthcare providers in developing infrastructure to support quality improvement activities. The chapter emphasizes the use of practice guidelines and protocols, computer-aided decision support, standardized performance measures, data feedback capabilities, and QI processes and resources. They particularly focused on systems quality improvement, which is critical for EMS, since EMS is involved in all phases of rural care, including triage, stabilization and transfer, and is part of many "handoffs" during patient encounters. The Committee on the Future of Rural Healthcare states:

> *An important role for rural providers is triage, stabilization and transfer of emergency cases. This process involves numerous "handoffs" that can negatively affect the timeliness of service delivery and provides an opportunity for miscommunication and medical errors. QI efforts need to focus on the continuum of care with special emphasis on these handoffs.*

However, for such a system to exist, much greater collaboration will be necessary among and between medical providers. True multidisciplinary workgroups must be employed to develop and implement, through consensus, protocols for emergency care services. Also, it must be recognized that in this new system, not all prehospital patient encounters will result in transfers. Thus, it is important that ambulance services be reimbursed for services rendered to patients who are not transferred to a hospital. As such, in addition to recommendations regarding

QI systems, payment reform recommendations are also included in this section. It is also important for the Federal government to ensure that existing rules do not unnecessarily stifle discussions among healthcare providers formally working on quality improvement efforts. Rule changes should be implemented to enhance communication among providers *during* emergencies as well as during discussions about *quality improvement.*

Related recommendations *from recent publications that relate to this topic*:

- Require performance improvement programs (including clinical quality and patient safety) at the hospital and community levels... [FPSP].
- Emphasize optimal interdisciplinary care of the ill or injured patient, including complex event management such as cardiac arrest and multiple casualty incidents [RFEMSA, Education Systems Chapter].
- Link/integrate EMS data systems with other relevant health information systems at all levels such as public health surveillance, crash, medical examiner, hospital discharge, and emergency department.... [RFEMSA, Information Systems Chapter].
- Encourage multi-system data collection for specific research and performance improvement purposes [RFEMSA, Information Systems Chapter].
- Fund the availability of training and toolkits to encourage effective local service/system quality improvement processes [RFEMSA, Evaluation Chapter].
- Ensure a mechanism for the on-going support and review of the NHTSA "Guide to Performance Measures" and "Leadership Guide to Quality Improvement for Emergency Medical Services Systems," and encourage their use in services and systems [RFEMSA, Evaluation Chapter].
- The Federal government should support the development of national standards for the following: emergency care performance measurement; categorization of all emergency care facilities; and protocols for the treatment, triage, and transport of prehospital patients [IOM-FEC EMS: *At the Crossroads*].
- The lead agency should strive for inclusiveness (all-facility and EMS system participation) by developing the process improvement program statewide.

This program should include facilities in the most remote areas of the State, for example, rural clinics and primary care centers in locations such as parks [MTSPE, Application of the Core Functions of Public Health to Trauma Systems Chapter].

- Implement the following Federal reimbursement reforms for emergency and interfacility EMS clinical care and operations: call-components performed by first-response, ALS intercept, ambulance, and other EMS response agencies that should be eligible for reimbursement (not duplicated on any given call) should include emergency response, assessment, treatment, triage, and transportation or other disposition that may, or may not, involve traditional transportation [RFEMSA, System Finance Chapter].
- The National Highway Traffic Safety Administration, in partnership with professional organizations, should convene a panel of individuals with multidisciplinary expertise to develop evidence-based model prehospital care protocols for the treatment, triage, and transport of patients [IOM-FEC EMS: *At the Crossroads*].
- The Centers for Medicare and Medicaid Services (CMS) should convene an *ad hoc* work group with expertise in emergency care, trauma, and EMS systems in order to evaluate the reimbursement of EMS and make recommendations regarding inclusion of readiness costs and permitting payment without transport [IOM-FEC EMS: *At the Crossroads*].
- The US Department of Health and Human Services should adopt rule changes to the Emergency Medical Treatment and Active Labor Act (EMTALA) and the Health Insurance Portability and Accountability Act (HIPAA) so that the original goals of the laws are preserved, but integrated systems may further develop [IOM-FEC *Hospital-Based: Emergency Care at the Breaking Point*].

Strategy III: Strengthening Human Resources

The IOM Committee on Rural Health recognized that human resources are critical assets in every rural community's efforts to enhance individual and population health and suggested that the current healthcare workforce is poorly prepared to "address the quality challenge."

The Committee recommended that:

Congress should provide appropriate resources...to expand experientially based workforce training program in rural areas to ensure that all healthcare professionals master the core competencies...

The Committee recognizes the following core competencies:

1) Providing patient-centered care;

2) Working in interdisciplinary teams;

3) Employing evidence-based practice;

4) Applying quality improvement methodologies; and

5) Utilizing informatics.

For *all* disciplines, the committee demanded changes to continuing education as well as new provider training programs and recommended increasing or enhancing experiential learning programs in rural environments, recruiting rural faculty and students, and expanding distance education.

The Committee on Rural Health, in discussing EMS education specifically, noted that the volunteer nature of rural EMS exacerbates the staffing challenges of rural ambulance services. It is a challenge to offer training programs that meet the needs of volunteers, who have limited time and may be reticent to drive long distances for education. With increasing reliance on two incomes in many rural households, volunteers may find it difficult to find the time necessary to devote to continuing education. Recognizing this, the Committee suggested that technology-based distance learning is the key to the future of EMS education. The Committee also recognized the importance of creative recruitment and retention strategies for rural America, but the report focused on recruitment/ retention strategies of medical professionals and overlooked any specific recommendations on EMS.

Other recently published policy documents have included extensive series of recommendations focused on a number of aspects of workforce development and enhancement. First, there are a group of recommendations that suggest the creation of tools and funding, to be deployed at the State and community level, to enhance recruitment and retention programs, including volunteer incentive programs which address the unique aspects of volunteer ambulance services that are common to America's rural areas.

Specific recommendations include:

- Foster the development of a culture of volunteerism and community service through local schools in partnership with community agencies [RFEMSA, Human Resources Chapter].
- Development of a national model to enhance career mobility within EMS practice levels, and between EMS and other health professions, to enhance the ability of rural/frontier areas to retain health workers who wish to gain new skills or advance or change healthcareers [RFEMSA, Education Systems Chapter].
- Recognition of the need for flexible scheduling to accommodate the lifestyle realities of rural volunteers [RFEMSA, Education Systems Chapter].

A second set of recommendations from these reports focus specifically on ways the education system must be structured to meet the needs of rural EMS professionals who need access to continuing education:

- Fund at the State and national levels a Rural/Frontier EMS Education and Training Initiative including·
  - funding to geographic areas which considers progress in completing community EMS assessments and informed self-determination processes;
  - funding through State EMS offices where needed, to develop effective systems of training and education program/system quality review and approval; and
  - development of flexible models for the implementation of a national model, including certificate and college-based programs, for providing basic, intermediate, and advanced EMS training and continuing education to rural/frontier areas and its implementation through State EMS offices [RFEMSA, Education Systems Chapter].

- Subsidization of training courses and continuing education programs and the instructor, equipment supply, and technical assistance infrastructure necessary to make them accessible to rural/frontier areas [RFEMSA, Education Systems Chapter].
- The use of interoperable systems of telemedicine and distance learning to improve the accessibility of training courses, effective quality improvement, and continuing education programs [RFEMSA, Education Systems Chapter].
- Incentives to increase the involvement of university medical centers and area health education centers to provide outreach educational programs to rural and frontier areas [RFESMA, Education Systems Chapter].
- Improved rural/frontier accessibility to training programs in emergency medical dispatch, critical incident stress management, and occupational safety training; as well as continuing education programs with curriculum content geared to rural/frontier application as appropriate [RFEMSA, Education Systems Chapter].
- Encouraging the development of realistic, dynamic patient simulators and mannequins for case-based and psychomotor skill training and critical decision-making improvement. Support for the development of patient simulator outreach programs [RFEMSA, Education Systems Chapter].
- The committee recommends that States link rural hospitals with academic health centers to enhance opportunities for professional consultation, telemedicine, patient referral and transport, and continuing professional education [IOM-FEC Hospital-Based: Emergency Care at the Breaking Point].
- Development of State/regional stockpiling, and sharing of expensive training devices such as mannequins and patient simulators [RFEMSA, Education Systems Chapter].
- Ongoing assessment by rural/frontier EMS agencies and local hospitals of their resources and needs, and searching for common educational opportunities [RFEMSA, Education Systems Chapter].
- The lead agency assists in ensuring a competent workforce through evaluation, training, and education and monitors the availability and

effectiveness of trauma systems [MTSPE, Application of the Core Functions of Public Health to Trauma Systems Chapter].

- States should strengthen the EMS workforce by requiring national accreditation of paramedic education programs, accepting national certification for State licensure, and adopting common EMS certification levels [IOM-FEC EMS: *At the Crossroads*].

A final group of recommendations specifically highlight the need for leadership and management training for both service chiefs and EMS medical directors. Ambulance service directors often rise "through the ranks" and are not trained to oversee the business of running an EMS service. Administrative aspects of running a service may be overlooked and poorly administered. Similarly, EMS medical directors very rarely receive training specific to their role of overseeing an ambulance service[s].

These recommendations are:

- A national EMS service leadership and service management training model should be developed and shared with all State, territorial and tribal governments. This model should include successful practices in EMS volunteer and paid human resources management [RFEMSA, Human Resources Chapter].
- Improved rural/frontier accessibility to a training program for service managers which includes EMS leadership, public and elected official advocacy, public education, grant-writing, data collection, research, governing board management, and volunteer management among other topics [RFEMSA, Education Systems Chapter].
- Ensuring the delivery of quality emergency medical services to rural populations is also complicated by the make up and skill level of prehospital EMS personnel, and associated issues of management, funding, and medical direction for rural EMS systems [IOM – FEC EMS: *At the Crossroads*].
- Prepare and protect rural/frontier emergency and primary care physicians to serve as EMS medical directors and assure adequate systems of performance improvement to support their activities [RFEMSA, Medical Oversight Chapter].

- Review all existing EMS medical oversight courses and establish a Rural/ Frontier EMS Medical Directors Course, which should be made available and distributed through multiple mechanisms to allow maximum access by EMS Medical Directors [RFEMSA, Medical Oversight Chapter].
- EMS medical oversight must be introduced in medical schools and included in the curriculums of primary care residency programs [RFEMSA, Medical Oversight Chapter].
- The committee believes that physicians who provide medical direction for EMS systems should meet standardized minimum requirements for training and certification that are reflective of their responsibilities [IOM-FEC EMS: *At the Crossroads*].

Strategy IV: Finance

Quality Through Collaboration stresses that payment systems must ensure the financial stability of rural healthcare systems in order to ensure that these systems can invest in human resources, information and communications technology, and quality improvement efforts. The report demands that "pilot" pay-for-performance systems must be tested with demonstration projects in rural areas to ensure these systems do not harm the rural healthcare delivery system.

Furthermore, they suggest that pay-for-performance systems for rural areas may need to involve linkages of several types of healthcare providers, which would most certainly include EMS. They also encourage rural healthcare providers to work collaboratively with other community leaders to develop community-wide initiatives aimed at improving health behaviors, with the goal of examining community health system effectiveness at addressing the quality aims of the IOM "Quality Chasm" series (safety, effectiveness, efficiency, patient-centeredness, timeliness, and equity).

Quality Through Collaboration discussed current funding for various health system sectors. For EMS, they noted that the majority of revenue is derived from transport fees, while the remainder of revenue comes from State and local taxes. The report notes that transport-based reimbursement is problematic for low-volume rural EMS providers whose costs are not necessarily linked to transport volume, but rather reflect the maintenance of a state of readiness.

Funding recommendations appearing in other key policy documents deal with several aspects of the financing of EMS. Several promote enhanced funding of State EMS offices to help them advance rural EMS issues. Others propose specific mechanisms through which local ambulance services would be more equitably reimbursed for the services they provide. These alternative payments systems would alleviate the financial strain imposed by a system that reimburses on the basis of transport and thus, does not reflect the cost of preparedness for low-volume rural ambulance services. Other recommendations encourage better access to grant funding, and specifically to preparedness funding. *The Rural and Frontier EMS Agenda for the Future* specifically implores CMS and other payors to reimburse rural EMS providers for a broad range of prevention and primary care services beyond emergency care. Authors of the *Agenda* recognize that declining populations in some remote areas will also result in declining numbers of health professionals. EMS is likely to be the last "link" in the healthcare safety net for many of these areas; paying cross-trained personnel with EMS training for preventive, primary care, and emergency services may be the only way to ensure access to care in the remote countryside.

Recommendations include:

- Adequately fund the State EMS lead agency to enable it to carry out its designated responsibilities [RFEMSA, Legislation and Regulation Chapter].
- Create funding incentives and legislation models to help State EMS lead agencies acquire sufficient legal basis, authority, resources, and leadership to broadly develop and implement EMS systems on an ongoing basis and to provide sufficient flexibility to adapt to the unique needs of rural/frontier EMS [RFEMSA, Legislation and Regulation Chapter].
- Implement the following Federal reimbursement reforms for emergency and interfacility EMS clinical care and operations [RFEMSA, System Finance Chapter]:
  - Call-components performed by first-response, ALS intercept, ambulance and other EMS response agencies that should be eligible for reimbursement (not duplicated on any given call) should include emergency response, assessment, treatment, triage, and transportation

or other disposition that may, or may not, involve traditional transportation.

- Retrospective review of medical necessity should not be done for emergency response calls.
- Immediately implement the patient condition codes model from the Negotiated Rule-Making process.
- Remove the "35 mile" restriction on cost-based reimbursement for EMS agencies that are owned and operated by Critical Access Hospitals.
- Employ definitions of "access" and "rural" (and its degrees) in reimbursement, which will help to maintain an adequate rural/frontier EMS infrastructure.
- Consider a "critical access ambulance service" definition or other means to ensure a minimal level of EMS infrastructure in all geographic areas.
- Ensure that interfacility transports that are "appropriate" from an EMTALA perspective are fairly reimbursed and not subjected to retrospective medical necessity determinations.
- Adopt reimbursement practices that encourage patient treatment and recovery at the facility closest to the patient's home that is desired by the patient and capable of providing the care required at the given stage of recovery.
- Facilitate the use of subscription services as a part of the overall funding of the EMS safety net infrastructure, in cooperation with State insurance authorities.
- Consider a single fiscal intermediary for all EMS providers, and develop a "successful practice" guide to assist EMS providers in maximizing billing efficiency and accuracy.

• Form and fund through county, regional, State or Federal tax dollars, rural/frontier EMS operational or service-contracting networks in those areas where they provide economies of scale, improved access to EMS care, improved quality and/or increased tax payer value [RFEMSA, System Finance Chapter].

- Make Federal and State domestic preparedness and response funding programs such as those of the US Department of Homeland Security, CDC, HRSA, and the Office for Domestic Preparedness (ODP) available explicitly and categorically to EMS systems and providers including private and for-profit agencies [RFEMSA, System Finance Chapter].
- CMS, MCOs and other third-party payers should fund EMS-based community healthcare pilot projects and define EMS personnel as reimbursement-eligible care-providers under physician medical oversight for primary care, prevention, and other services they render [RFEMSA, System Finance Chapter].
- The goal of trauma system financing is to provide the public with a consistent, reliable, and readily available healthcare safety net for injured patients [MTSPE, System Finance Chapter].
- Financial resources are needed to support the EMS system response for trauma care. Funds are needed to train EMS personnel to care for injured individuals. Although some EMS providers volunteer their time to care for injured patients, in many locations, salary support must be included in financial planning. Financial support for a medical director to provide oversight, protocols for care, and performance improvement guidance is required. Local EMS agencies also must have the resources for ambulances, as well as the equipment and supplies for patient care [MTSPE, System Finance Chapter].
- Funding should be increased for the emergency medical component of preparedness – both EMS and hospital-based – especially for personal protective equipment, training, and planning [IOM-FEC EMS: *At the Crossroads*].
- To determine whether incentives are properly aligned, CMS should investigate whether Medicare and Medicaid payment methodologies should be revised to support payment for emergency care services in the most appropriate setting (including treat and release) [IOM-FEC EMS: *At the Crossroads*].

Strategy V: Building an Information and Communication Technology (ICT) Infrastructure

The IOM Committee on the Future of Rural Health believes information and communication technology is a powerful tool that has great potential to produce improvements in the quality of patient care. The committee recognizes that there are key issues and challenges for rural providers to develop the necessary infrastructure to support a "paperless" healthcare system, and they advance recommendations to help address these issues.

Where does EMS fit into this discussion? With current discussions emphasizing the use of telemedicine, electronic health records, electronic bedside physician order entry systems, e-prescribing, etc., it may not be readily apparent how EMS providers might benefit from this transition to a paperless system. The IOM suggests several possibilities, however. For example, they discuss studies of cardiac emergencies where data transfer capabilities allowed physicians to monitor electrocardiograms during prehospital care to assess the need for administration of thrombolytics. Another recent study found benefits in the use of abdominal sonography for prehospital care. A Vermont study found benefit in linking trauma surgeons to rural emergency departments via videoconferencing in the initial treatment of trauma patients. These studies suggest important benefits for rural EMS in developing more advanced information and communications technologies to support prehospital patient care. In fact, the *Rural and Frontier EMS Agenda for the Future* and the IOM *Future of Emergency Care* explored an even broader range of information technology issues. One focus was the enhanced use of telemedicine and interactive media for distance learning. A second theme was technology to enhance emergency notification, including systems such as 9-1-1, crash notification systems, and home monitoring technologies. A third theme was enhanced interoperable communication systems, and a fourth was the use of EMS information systems for enhanced evaluation and performance improvement purposes, as well as public health surveillance purposes.

Recommendations include:

- Recognition [within the education model] that EMS education will be provider-need specific, conducted with varied teaching techniques emphasizing hands-on training, and (where appropriate) distance learning to assist the transfer of learning and retention of essential skills and knowledge so as to provide state-of-the-art rural emergency care [RFEMSA, Education Systems Chapter].

- The use of interoperable systems of telemedicine and distance learning to improve the accessibility of training courses, effective quality improvement, and continuing education programs [RFEMSA, Education Systems Chapter].
- A variety of learning methods should be used. Web-based learning opportunities that can be later archived are one cost-effective way to educate a large number of persons [MTSPE, Application of the Core Functions of Public Health to Trauma Systems Chapter].
- Ensure telephonic or other access to completed Enhanced 9-1-1 (i.e., including accurate physical addressing) and Wireless Enhanced 9-1-1 (i.e., with geolocation of the calling device) through effective Federal and State programs, mandates and funding [RFEMSA, Public Access Chapter].
  - State EMS offices should consider a patient-centered, medical leadership initiative to encourage E-9-1-1 and WE-9-1-1 system completion where other approaches have failed.
  - Federal funding for State and local public safety communications development should consider progress toward E-9-1-1 and WE-9-1-1 systems completion.
- Integrate Automatic Crash Notification (and other Intelligent Transportation System and Department of Defense technology) and health event advice lines into the process of EMS public access and EMS resource deployment [RFEMSA, Public Access Chapter].
- States should establish formal plans for roadside call-box, satellite, and/or cellular networks to effectively cover all rural/frontier primary roads [RFEMSA, Public Access Chapter].
- As home health monitoring devices and automated remote diagnostic technology develop, EMS leaders should pursue roles for EMS in their

use to further EMS-based community health services [RFEMSA, Public Access Chapter].

- Conduct comprehensive State EMS communication needs assessments upon which to base Federal, State, and local investment in communications infrastructure improvement [RFEMSA, Communication Systems Chapter].
- The Universal Service Program fund, Federal Communications Commission, frequency allocation and other national public safety communications organizations and agencies should work to assure that rural/frontier EMS communications are enhanced [RFEMSA, Communication Systems Chapter].
- Re-dedicate radio spectrum to EMS and other public safety use [RFEMSA, Communication Systems Chapter].
- Explore EMS applications of innovative communications and resource management technologies. Encourage Federal and State agencies to provide pilot funding and access to their agencies' technology developers and resources for this purpose [RFEMSA, Communication Systems Chapter].
- EMS leaders should continue to develop ongoing paths of communication with State and Federal telecommunications interoperability and Intelligent Transportation Systems industry planning entities [RFEMSA, Communication Systems Chapter].
- Implement and maintain a local EMS information system at every local EMS service/agency. Maintain data on every EMS event in a manner which is timely and able to drive the quality of the EMS system service and patient care delivery [RFEMSA, Information Systems Chapter].
- Link/integrate EMS data systems with other relevant health information systems at all levels such as public health surveillance, crash, medical examiner, hospital discharge, and emergency department, including CDC surveillance monitoring systems [RFEMSA, Information Systems Chapter].
- The following information technologies could significantly enhance emergency care: (1) dashboard systems that track and coordinate patient flow; (2) communications systems that enable ED physicians to link to patients' records or providers; (3) clinical decision-support programs that

improve decision-making; (4) documentation systems for collecting and storing patient data; (5) computerized training and information retrieval; and (6) systems to facilitate public health surveillance. Given their demonstrated effectiveness in the emergency care setting, the committee recommends that hospitals adopt robust information and communications systems to improve the safety and quality of emergency care and enhance hospital efficiency. The committee recognizes that the appropriate prioritization of and investment in these approaches will vary based on each institution's resources and needs [IOM-FEC Hospital-Based Emergency Care: At the Breaking Point].

- The trauma Management Information System (MIS) is used to facilitate ongoing assessment and assurance of system performance and outcomes and provides a basis for continuously improving the trauma system including a cost-benefit analysis [MTSPE, Application of the Core Functions of Public Health to Trauma Systems Chapter].
- Communications among EMS, public safety, public health, and other hospital providers is even more problematic given the technical challenges associated with developing interoperable networks. As a result of these challenges and the need for improved coordination, the committee recommends that hospitals, trauma centers, EMS agencies, public safety departments, emergency management offices, and public health agencies develop integrated and interoperable communications and data systems [IOM FEC EMS: *At the Crossroads*].
- Nevertheless, the use of telemedicine and distance learning allows previously inaccessible training to penetrate remote areas and new, more realistic and dynamic patient simulators to allow case-based honing of critical skills and decision-making [IOM-FEC: EMS: *At the Crossroads*].
- The development of Automatic Crash Notification (ACN) technology, now becoming more widely available, has further improved emergency response, providing immediate and increasingly detailed crash information to dispatchers automatically, even before anyone on scene places a call [IOM-FEC EMS: *At the Crossroads*].

Conclusion: Rural Health and Emergency Medical Services – Shared Goals

The Institute of Medicine charged their Committee on the Future of Rural Health with recommending priority objectives and identifying changes in polices and programs to enhance the quality of care in rural areas.

The IOM similarly charged their Committee on the Future of Emergency Care in the US Health System with developing recommendations to improve the emergency care system in this country.

Developers of the *Rural and Frontier EMS Agenda for the Future* specifically addressed the bridge between rural health and EMS, noting that EMS must be integrated into the broader rural health system.

The Model Trauma System Planning and Evaluation Document explicitly linked the trauma system and public health.

The staff of the Office of Rural Health Policy's Rural Hospital Flexibility Program has created a set of recommendations designed to influence program development, primarily within States, through the Rural Hospital Flexibility (FLEX) Program, which has a focus on rural health issues including EMS.

It is likely that all of the stakeholders from these various groups envisioned that their recommendations would influence policy-making and funding allocations at local, State and Federal levels. Indeed, many stakeholders are developing strategies to implement recommendations outlined in these respective documents.

The intended value of the "crosswalk" of these recent publications is to highlight how much common ground exists among a broad-based and influential set of providers, policy-makers, and other stakeholders with interests in rural and frontier EMS.

An incredibly diverse array of stakeholders participated in the development of these key documents. Some groups that have not been specifically highlighted earlier in this report are the National Association of State EMS Officials (the key association linking State EMS programs at a national level), the National

Organization of State Offices of Rural Health (the national organization representing all 50 State rural health offices), the Rural EMS & Trauma Technical Assistance Center, and the National Rural Health Association. Clearly, a diverse and broad-based set of stakeholders is currently engaged in policy discussions about the future of rural EMS and trauma care. This synergy is exciting and suggests that the time is right for advocates and policy-makers to pursue a common strategy to ensure a bright future for rural and frontier EMS in this country.

APPENDIX A

References/List of Key Documents

The following is a list of key documents published in the last 3 years that formed the basis for this comparative report.

1) Institute of Medicine of the National Academies (2005). *Quality Through Collaboration: The Future of Rural Health.* Washington, DC: The National Academies Press. *www.nap.edu*

As part of a Institute of Medicine quality initiative, the IOM produced two reports, *To Err is Human: Building a Safer Health System and Crossing the Quality Chasm: A New Health System for the 21st Century.* These reports highlighted serious problems with the overall quality of care delivered in the United States. *Quality Through Collaboration* is part of a third phase of the IOM's quality initiative focused on operationalizing the vision of a future health system described in the *Quality Chasm* report.

2) McGinnis, K.K. (2004). *Rural and Frontier EMS Agenda for the Future.* Kansas City, MO: National Rural Health Association.

Funded by the Office of Rural Health Policy, this document was the result of a consensus-building process overseen by the National Association of EMS Officials and the National Organization of State Offices of Rural Health. Comments were accepted from around the country through an interactive website and a national consensus meeting in a process lasting a little over 1 year. The purpose was to create a vision for rural EMS, building upon the seminal work of the National Highway Traffic Safety Administration's 1996 *EMS Agenda for the Future.*

3) Health Resources and Services Administration, Office of Rural Health Policy. *Rural Hospital Flexibility Program Strategic Plan.*

The Rural Hospital Flexibility Program is a Federal initiative that provides funding to State governments to strengthen rural health. The program allows small hospitals the flexibility to reconfigure operations and be licensed as Critical

Access Hospitals (CAHs), offers cost-based reimbursement for Medicare acute inpatient and outpatient services to CAHs, encourages the development of rural health networks, and provides annual grants to State Offices of Rural Health to help implement a CAH program in the context of broader initiatives to strengthen the rural healthcare infrastructure. The strategic objectives of the program are outlined in a strategic plan. The plan can be found online at *http://ruralhealth.hrsa.gov/funding/FlexStratPlan.asp*

4) Institute of Medicine of the National Academies (2006). *Future of Emergency Care: Hospital-Based Emergency Care.* Washington, DC: The National Academies Press. *www.nap.edu*

The Institute of Medicine's Committee on the Future of Emergency Care in the United States Health System was convened in 2003 to examine the state of emergency care in the United States; to create a vision for the future of emergency care, including trauma care; and to make recommendations to help the Nation achieve that vision. Their findings and recommendations are presented in three reports. One report, *Hospital-Based Emergency Care: At the Breaking Point*, explores the changing role of the hospital emergency department and describes the national epidemic of overcrowded emergency departments and trauma centers.

5) Institute of Medicine of the National Academies (2006). *Future of Emergency Care: Emergency Care for Children: Growing Pains.* Washington, DC: The National Academies Press. *www.nap.edu*

The Institute of Medicine's Committee on the Future of Emergency Care in the United States Health System was convened in 2003 to examine the state of emergency care in the US, to create a vision for the future of emergency care, including trauma care, and to make recommendations to help the Nation achieve that vision. The second report, *Emergency Care for Children: Growing Pains,* describes the unique challenges of emergency care for children.

6) Institute of Medicine of the National Academies (2006). *Future of Emergency Care: Emergency Medical Services at the Crossroads.* Washington, DC: The National Academies Press. *www.nap.edu*

The Institute of Medicine's Committee on the Future of Emergency Care in the United States Health System was convened in 2003 to examine the state of emergency care in the United States, to create a vision for the future of emergency care, including trauma care, and to make recommendations to help the Nation achieve that vision.

The third report, *Emergency Medical Services At the Crossroads,* describes the development of EMS systems over the last 40 years and the fragmented system that exists today.

7) US Department of Health and Human Services, Health Resources and Services Administration (2006). *Model Trauma System Planning and Evaluation.*

This document was developed through a collaborative process involving an incredible array of professional organizations and Federal agencies. It is a guide to modern state-wide trauma system development. Its purpose is to provide trauma care professionals, public health officials, and healthcare policy experts with the direction to use the public health approach, a scientifically proven method, when developing and evaluating trauma systems. Extensive information on the model can be found online at *http://www.hrsa.gov/trauma/model.htm*

APPENDIX B

Acknowledgements

Data for the statistical analysis component of this study was made available by the National Registry of EMTs (NREMT), who approved the plan of analysis December 13, 2005. We would like to extend a special thanks to the Longitudinal EMT Attributes and Demographics Study (LEADS) committee. Without access to the LEADS survey data, this study would not have been possible.

This compendium was made possible by funds provided by ORHP and the Rural Emergency Medical Services and Trauma Technical Assistance Center (REMSTTAC), and the Kansas Department of Health & Environment (KDHE)-Office of Local & Rural Health. Special thanks for producing this compendium go to KDHE-Office of Local & Rural Health staff, Chris Tilden, Interim Director and to REMSTTAC staff, Nels Sanddal, Director; Heather Soucy, Program Support Specialist; Teri Sanddal, Associate Director and Joe Hansen, Assistant Director and members of the Policy Document Workgroup at REMSTTAC.

Nels D Sanddal, M S, REMT-B, Co-chair
Director
Rural Emergency Medical Services and Trauma Technical Assistance Center.

Chris Tilden, Ph.D., Co-chair
Director
Kansas Department of Health & Environment
Office of Local & Rural Health.

Contributors and Reviewers:

Thomas J Esposito, MD, MPH, FACS
Medical Director, REMSTTAC
Professor & Chief Section of Trauma
Surgery
Department of Surgery
Loyola University Medical Center.

Joe Hansen, Associate Director
Rural Emergency Medical Services and
Trauma Technical Assistance Center.

Tami Lichtenberg, TASC Program
Manager
Rural Health Resource Center
Technical Assistance and Services Center.

Jerry Overton, Executive Director
Richmond Ambulance Authority.

Jacob Rueda, Project Officer
US Department of Health and Human Services
Health Resources and Services
Administration
Office of Rural Health Policy.

Gary Wingrove, Technical Consultant
Technical Assistance and Services Center
Rural Health Resource Center.

APPENDIX C

REMSTTAC Stakeholders Group

Katrina Altenhofen, MPH, REMT-B
State Coordinator
Emergency Medical Services of for Children
Iowa Department of Public Health.

Jane W Ball, RN, DrPH
Executive Director (Retired)
EMSC National Resource Center
Trauma-EMS Technical Assistance Center.

Bethany Cummings, DO
Rural Affairs Ad Hoc Committee
National Association of EMS Physicians.

Drew Dawson, Chief, EMS Division
National Highway Traffic Safety
Administration.

Tom Esposito, MD
Medical Director
Rural EMS and Trauma Technical
Assistance Center.

Blanca Fuertes, Past Project Officer
US Department of Health and Human Services
Health Resources and Services
Administration
Office of Rural Health Policy.

Christian L Hanna, MPH
Michigan Public Health Institute
Child and Adolescent Health.

Bob Heath, EMS Education Coordinator
Nevada State Health Division
Intermountain Regional EMS for Children
Coordinating Council.

Marilyn Jarvis
Assistant Director for Continuing
Education
Extended University
Montana State University.

Douglas F Kupas, MD
Rural Affairs Ad Hoc Committee
National Association of EMS Physicians.

Fergus Laughridge, Program Manager
Nevada State Health Division
EMS Bureau of Licensure & Certification.

Tami Lichtenberg, Program Manager
Technical Assistance and Services Center
Rural Health Resource Center.

Tommy Loyacono, MPA
National Association of Emergency
Medical Technicians.

Patrick Malone, Director
Initiative for Rural Emergency Medical Services
University of Vermont.

N Clay Mann, PhD, MS
Center Director of Research
Professor of Pediatrics
Intermountain Injury Control Research Center
University of Utah.

Evan Mayfield, MS
US Department of Health and Human Services
Center for Disease Control Office of the Commissioner.

Charity G Moore, PhD
Research Assistant Professor
Cecil G. Sheps Center for Health Services Research
University of North Carolina at Chapel Hill.

Carol Miller, Executive Director
National Center for Frontier Communities.

Kimberly K. Obbink, M.Ed, Director
Extended University
Montana State University
Jerry Overton, Executive Director
Richmond Amublance Authority.

Daniel Patterson, PhD
AHRQ-NRSA Post-Doctoral Research Fellow
Cecil G. Sheps Center for Health Services Research
University of North Carolina at Chapel Hill.

Davis Patterson, PhD, Research Scientist
Battelle Centers for Public Health
Research and Evaluation.

Ana Maria Puente, Past Project Officer
US Department of Health and Human Services
Health Resources and Services
Administration
International Health/Office of Rural Health Policy.

Jacob L Rueda III, PhD, Project Officer
US Department of Health and Human Services
Health Resources and Services
Administration
Office of Rural Health Policy.

Kristine Sande, Project Director
Rural Assistance Center
University of North Dakota Center for Rural Health.

Mary Sheridan, Director
State Offices of Rural Health
Idaho Department of Health and Welfare.

Dan Summers, RN, BSN, CEN, EMT-P
Director of Education
Center for Rural Emergency Medicine
West Virginia University.

Chris Tilden, PhD, Director
Kansas Department of Health & Environment
Office of Local & Rural Health.

Robert K. Waddell II
Secretary/Treasurer
National Association of EMS Educators.

Bill White, President
National Native American EMS Association.

Gary Wingrove, Technical Consultant
Technical Assistance and Services Center
Rural Health Resource Center.

Jill Zabel Myers, Healthcare Consulting
Wipfli LLP.

8

Rural Health Insurance – Rising to the Challenge

This article is focused on the challenges of rural health insurance in China and documents some responses at the government level. Rising to the challenge, China's government recently developed plans for a New Cooperative Medical Scheme (NCMS). The new county level scheme has also been initiated against a background of an almost total collapse of the old village-level rural Cooperative Medical Scheme (CMS). Both the programs face challenges relating to breadth and depth of coverage, cost control, quality assurance and so on. China's central government has also seen increases in its tax revenues, and is committed to spending some of them on rural health in general and on the NCMS in particular.

Background to the Briefing Note

How can health insurance coverage in China be expanded and deepened? How can health insurers keep costs down and ensure high quality care for their members? What role should government have in health insurance in China? These were some of the questions addressed by two critical reviews of the Chinese-language and English-language literatures on rural and urban health insurance in China and abroad.*

The reviews come at a key moment. Against a background of an almost total collapse of the old rural Cooperative Medical Scheme (CMS) and declining coverage in urban areas, the government has started piloting a new CMS in over 300 counties and is looking to extend coverage of the newly reformed urban scheme. Both programs face challenges relating to breadth and depth of coverage, cost control, quality assurance, and so on.

This Briefing Note focuses for the most part on the rural health insurance challenge. It traces the changes in the 1990s in coverage, explores the problems that are likely to be encountered as the government's new rural health insurance program is rolled out, and suggests that the solutions to many of these problems lie in the experiences of the past—both in the rural and urban schemes.

The Legacy of Economic Liberalization – Falling and Shallower Coverage

Under China's pre-reform planned economy, almost all citizens were covered by some form of health insurance. Agricultural workers were covered by the old commune-based CMS, State-Owned Enterprise (SOE) workers were covered by the Labor Insurance Scheme (LIS), and civil servants and other government workers were covered by the Government Insurance Scheme (GIS). There were some gaps in coverage (not all urban schemes covered dependents, for example), but the gaps were relatively small (during the 1970s the CMS covered an estimated 90% of the rural population). China's near-universal coverage is thought to have been one reason for its spectacular success in improving health outcomes during the 1970s.[1]

* This briefing note was prepared as part of the World Bank's (WB) ongoing study on China's rural health sector. The study—referred to as the *China Rural Health AAA* (Analytical and Advisory Activities)—is being undertaken in collaboration with the Ministry of Health (MOH) and other government agencies, as well as with selected international partners. The reviews upon which this briefing note is based were prepared by two teams, comprising Professors Wen Chen of Fudan University, Gordon Liu of Peking University, Brian Nolan of the Economic and Social Research Institute (Ireland), Mao Zhengzhong Of China West Medical University, and Liu Yuanli of Harvard University. The team benefited from the comments of Wang Hufeng of the Ministry of Labor and Social Security and Han Jun of the State Council Development Research Center, who were the discussants for these critical reviews at the AAA workshop in July 2004. The briefing note was prepared by the World Bank AAA team. The findings, interpretations, and conclusions expressed herein are those of the authors, and do not necessarily reflect the views of the World Bank or those of its Executive Directors or the governments they represent. For further information on the China Rural Health AAA and related activities, contact L Richard Meyers (*lmeyers@worldbank.org*).

China's transition from a planned to a market economy from 1980 onwards brought dramatic reductions in health insurance coverage. The decollectivization of agriculture resulted in an almost total collapse of the CMS. By 1993 less than 10% of the rural population had health insurance (Figure 1). The mid-late 1990s saw several attempts to resuscitate the CMS.† Despite these initiatives, CMS coverage nationally remained stubbornly low. By 2003, 80% of China's rural population—some 640 million people—lacked health insurance (Figure 1). Half of the rural respondents in the 2003 NHS who said they had insurance said they were covered by either private (i.e., commercial) insurance or 'other' insurance.‡

Figure 1: Health Insurance Coverage in China has been Falling

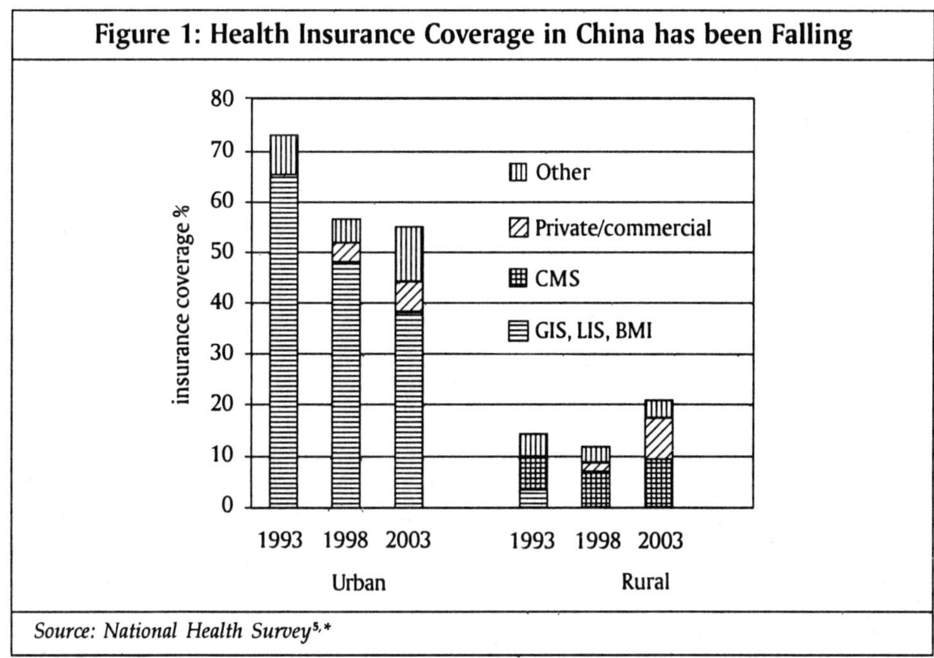

Source: National Health Survey[5,*]

† These included the RAND Sichuan CMS experiment in mid-1990s[2], the WHO 14 county study in the early 1990s[3], the UNICEF 10-county study in 1997-2000, the World Bank Health VIII project in the late 1990s, and the Harvard 2-county study in 2003[4].

‡ Examples of schemes in these categories would include schemes intended to provide broad coverage, as well as those targeted to specific groups, such as school children, where the risks covered are very limited. Little has been written about such schemes, even in the national media, and it is striking that they provide some form of coverage for as many as 10% of China's rural population.

* Figures for urban 2003 are from Ling Xu's presentation at December 2004 MOH seminar on the 2003 NHS survey. Figures for rural 2003 are from Main Findings from the 3rd NHS Survey, *www.moh.gov.cn*, accessed on April 21st, 2005.

Coverage in China's cities has also declined, though less dramatically than in rural areas. As China transitioned to a market economy, the SOE—the backbone of the LIS—came under increasing pressure. LIS coverage fell, as did GIS coverage. By 1998 nearly half the urban population lacked insurance coverage. A variety of reforms have been introduced, including the setting up in 1998 of a new single urban scheme known as Basic Medical Insurance (BMI), into which LIS and GIS are gradually being subsumed (Box 1). Despite these reforms, coverage by GIS/LIS/BMI continued to fall between 1998 and 2003. Had it not been for the growth of private and 'other' insurance schemes, coverage would have fallen below 40% in 2003.

Box 1: Urban Health Insurance Reform

Urban health insurance reform in China can be broken down into four phases.[6-8]

1988-94. Small-scale and preliminary reforms were introduced in a few cities, focusing primarily on the application of demand-side cost-sharing mechanisms under the existing GIS and LIS.

1995-98. Central government launched a formal pilot experiment of new community-based insurance models in the cities of Zhenjiang and Jiujiang. This pilot model introduced some fundamental changes in the existing GIS and LIS. The most significant changes included the socialization of financing, jointly contributed by employers and employees, to form a citywide insurance pool across all work units. The pooled funds were then distributed into individual Medical Savings Accounts (MSA) and a Social Pooling Account (SPA). In the end of 1996, the experiment reform was extended to 57 other cities.

1998-2003. In December 1998 a nationwide effort was called for by the State Council to reform the existing GIS and LIS in the remaining cities following the Zhenjiang and Jiujiang pilots. By the end of 2003, the vast majority of large cities had implemented the new Basic Medical Insurance (BMI) insurance program, covering over 109 million urban employees.

2000-present. In parallel to the above reforms, the government started to reform the hospital and pharmacy markets in an effort to lower costs or at least reduce inflation in the health sector.

It is not just the *number* of people covered by health insurance that has been falling. The *depth* of coverage has also been declining (Figure 2). By 1997, insured patients were paying more than *one third* of their inpatient costs out of their own pockets.[9] The falling depth of coverage reflected in part the introduction of formal cost containment measures but also the fact that in the transition to the market economy, many SOEs found it increasingly difficult to honor their LIS commitments. The government increasingly withdrew from its role of payer of last resort.[10] In Zhenjiang, for example, it was estimated that more than half of the SOEs were unable to fully reimburse the medical bills for their employees. The new schemes that have emerged also appear to be less generous than the old ones (Figure 2).

Figure 2: Inpatient Care Reimbursement Rates for the Insured have been Falling

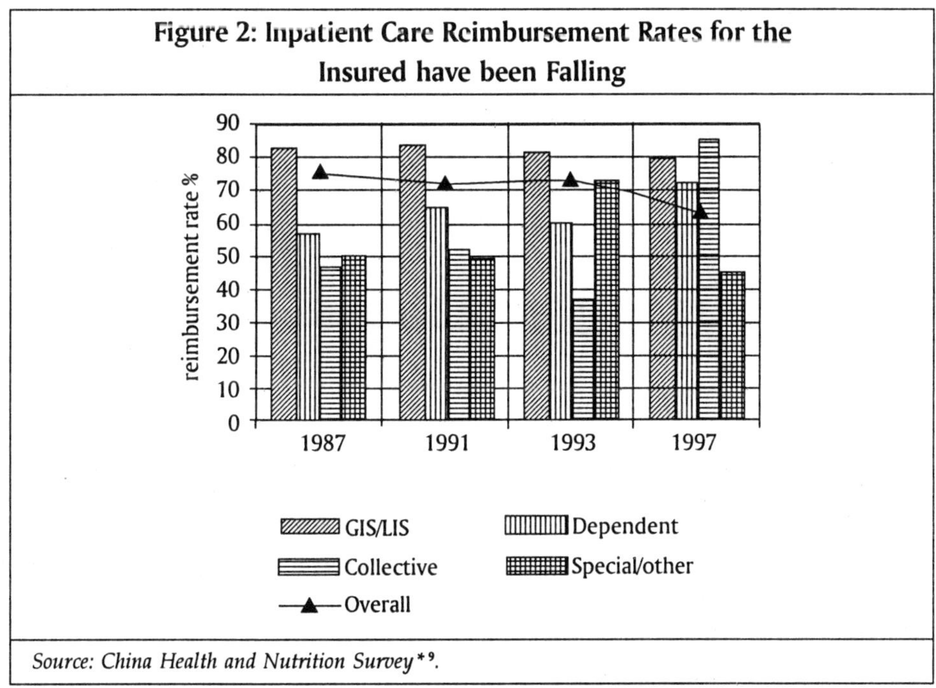

*Source: China Health and Nutrition Survey** [9].

Rising to the Rural Health Insurance Challenge – The Government's New CMS

While extending health insurance cover to China's 155 million uninsured urban residents is also an important task, a larger and—in the government's eyes—more urgent challenge is that of extending cover to China's 640 million rural uninsured. It is this that is the main focus of the remainder of the Briefing Note.

Rising to this challenge, China's government recently developed plans for a New Coperative Medical Scheme (NCMS). The scheme is currently being piloted in over 300 of China's more than 2000 counties, and will be rolled out to the rest of the country by 2010.

* The figures refer to actual reimbursement rates, not rates promised by the schemes. The CHNS is not statistically representative of the Chinese population but does cover a broad spectrum of China's provinces. The 'other' category is used in the CHNS as a catch-all for categories other than those listed explicitly in the questionnaire.

The NCMS differs from the old CMS in several important respects. Contributions from households—starting at 10 RMB per person, and to be paid on a voluntary basis—will be supplemented by a subsidy of 10 RMB or more from local government and a 10 RMB matching subsidy from central government in the case of households living in the poorer central and western provinces. The NCMS will operate at the county level rather than at the village or township level as was the case in the old CMS. In the pilots so far, enrolment is reported to be around 70%.

As the government rolls out the NCMS, it will encounter many challenges. As it does so, the government could usefully learn from relevant experiences in China—the various attempts of the 1990s to resuscitate CMS and the reforms of China's urban health insurance scheme—as well as experiences abroad.

Is the New CMS Affordable?

Can each of the parties realistically be expected to be able to afford their contribution of 10 RMB or more per person? Some have expressed doubts.

It would seem reasonable to expect central government to be able to afford its 10 RMB per resident of the central and western provinces. Central government spending on health is relatively small, as is total government spending on health by international standards. China's central government has also seen increases in its tax revenues, and is committed to spending some of them on rural health in general and on the NCMS in particular.

Whether local governments can afford their 10 RMB is less clear. The bulk of health spending in China is financed by local governments who are highly dependent on their own revenues. As a result, government spending per capita varies considerably across provinces—and even more so across counties. The more of the 10 RMB that counties have to finance rather than cities/prefectures and provinces, the more regressive the local government element of the NCMS cost will be. For poor counties, even 4 RMB per person could represent a fairly large fraction of their existing health spending. And the NCMS initiative comes at a bad time for local government officials. China is in the process of abolishing several agricultural taxes, which is reducing the tax revenues of townships and counties.

To some degree this is being offset by a shifting of expenditure responsibilities to higher levels and by the provision of compensating transfers, but these will go only part of the way to restoring township and county government revenues. This all assumes the 10 RMB contribution will be *additional* money—it may be that some local governments see the NCMS as an opportunity to shift from supply-side to demand-side subsidies.

The household contribution of 10 RMB or more seems affordable at least for the average household, given that it represents just 0.4% of the rural per capita income. It will, it is true, be a much larger fraction for poor households. However, this could be tackled by having the Ministry of Civil Affairs' Medical Assistance (MA) scheme help the poorest households with their NCMS contributions and perhaps their copayments too.*

The Benefit Package of the NCMS and its Effect on Enrolment

The key issue from the perspective of households is not whether they are *able* to pay 10 RMB but rather whether they are *willing* to pay it. Is NCMS a good buy for Chinese households? People's willingness to participate in the new CMS is likely to depend on a number of factors. But one key one is *how the benefits offered compare to the 10 RMB contribution.*

One important number to keep in mind is that 30 RMB per capita represents less than 20% of per capita annual health spending in rural areas. So, NCMS is going to leave a lot of expenses uncovered. It is important that the actuaries developing the NCMS benefit package do their arithmetic carefully. If they promise too much, the NCMS will quickly go bankrupt.

One option is to provide generous coverage (i.e., have low coinsurance rates) on low-frequency high-cost medical events—the sort that lead to 'catastrophic' medical expenses. One risk with this is that since very few people experience such expenses, most members will receive little *direct* financial assistance from the CMS. Of course, they receive *indirect* assistance since the CMS has reduced if not eliminated their exposure to the risk of catastrophic medical costs. But they may not see it that way. Potentially this attitude could be changed through education and social marketing.

* The links between health safety nets and the NCMS are to be discussed in a future Briefing Note on health safety nets.

But there is a further problem with a scheme that focuses exclusively on catastrophic costs, namely that people may delay seeking medical care until the problem becomes so severe that the care they need is serious enough for them to receive some assistance from the CMS. This happens in other countries, and there is no reason to think it wouldn't happen in China too. It may be better, therefore, to have a benefit package that covers both high-cost and low-cost events, and outpatient and inpatient care. The coinsurance rates ought to be higher for outpatient than inpatient care.

Should public health services such as immunization be covered by NCMS? There are those who say yes, on the grounds that they are under-funded and including them in the NCMS benefit package could help strengthen their provision. But there are also those who argue no, on the grounds that doing so would lead to additional claims of an already tight NCMS budget. Internationally, insurers have a mixed record on public health activities, not least because they tend to focus on their members and overlook the benefits of public health activities that accrue to non-members. The emerging practice seems to be to take public health programs and the financing of them *outside* the health insurance sector.

With less than 20% of average spending covered by NCMS, many households may feel the scheme does too little to reduce exposure to medical-expense risk. In that case, support for the NCMS may dwindle, and people will either not join or start to disenrol. If, as is likely, it is the 'better' risks (the young and healthy) who leave first, the NCMS will start making a loss, and contributions may need to be raised. This may prompt a further exodus by good risks, and a downward spiral will start, with the scheme eventually collapsing—a problem known as *adverse selection.*

The experience from other countries indicates that adverse selection can quickly undermine and ultimately precipitate the collapse of a purely voluntary scheme. *This does not depend on how sound the benefit package is from an actuarial standpoint, or on the fraction of average spending covered by the scheme.* It simply reflects the fact that in any population, there will be good risks and bad risks, and if the scheme is voluntary, the better risks will prefer to self-insure. It is for this reason that health insurance in industrialized countries is almost always compulsory.

Trustworthy and Competent Management – Key Ingredients of NCMS Success

It is not just a question of getting the NCMS benefit package right. There is another important lesson from the previous attempts to resuscitate CMS, especially in the UNICEF 10-county study, namely that *people need to trust the organizers of a CMS scheme if they are to participate in it.*

Trust is partly about eliminating corruption. Many CMS schemes that have failed have done so because of corruption. Involving beneficiaries in overseeing the CMS may help reduce corruption. This is one of the ideas underlying an experiment sponsored by Harvard University in Kaiyang county (Guizhou) and Zhenan county (Shaanxi), where villagers serve on the CMS board of directors.[4]

Some argue that the lack of trust in the resuscitated CMS schemes was sometimes due to management team members having a dual function as manager of an insurance fund and manager of a health facility. This led CMS members to wonder whether the CMS was acting in the interests of providers or CMS members. The fact that NCMS is to be located at county level and separate from the provider network should substantially militate against this. NCMS seems set to play the role of 'purchaser' for its members, negotiating service delivery arrangements—cost, quality, timing and location of treatment, etc.—on behalf of its members.

This calls for a strong NCMS management—one that is not simply trustworthy but also capable of discharging the functions of an insurer-purchaser agency. This will require building up a professional staff, albeit one that is overseen by local representatives.

The task of developing competent management in NCMS is a challenging one, as comparisons with BMI indicate. BMI typically covers about 10,000 members at the county level, albeit with a more generous benefit package. Each county might have as many as 15 full-time staff. NCMS, by contrast, is expected to cover an average of 250,000 members per county, and is also more complex in many respects. Its members are likely to be more heterogeneous in terms of their health conditions and geographical locations than BMI members. NCMS involves a more complex fund-collection process than the BMI, where contributions are collected through a payroll tax. NCMS also has to deal with a more diverse set of providers.

One question for NCMS management to answer is: Which providers will be certified to deliver care at the NCMS's expense? This process is critical for holding down NCMS costs as well as ensuring NCMS members receive quality care. But it is also critical to ensuring access. Will village doctors be certified even though they are private? Will only public township hospitals be certified? Restricting the list to public providers may have has some merit but has the disadvantage that people may find they cannot use their usual provider with their NCMS coverage. This may mean households have to travel further to see a provider than before. It may also mean that NCMS results in households simply substituting public visits for private visits, rather than increasing the overall number of visits.

Central government could play a useful role in helping develop trustworthy and competent management in the NCMS, providing technical assistance, and ensuring that there is learning from and cooperation with relevant parts of government, such as BMI, tax bureaux, and so on.

Moral Hazard and NCMS Costs

In the rush to extend coverage to China's large rural uninsured population, one further important lesson needs to be kept firmly in mind. It is a lesson that comes from China's own experience with urban health insurance in the 1980s and 1990s. And it is one that comes through loud and clear from other countries, especially the United States. The lesson is that *health insurance is associated with a problem known as moral hazard.*

This curious term refers to the fact that with someone else picking up the bill for treatment, patients and providers alike have an incentive to increase the amount of care delivered—extra tests, more expensive medicines, a switch to surgery even though it is not medically necessary, and so on.

China's experience with urban health insurance illustrates this nicely. LIS and GIS members paid very little out of their own pockets, and providers were paid on a fee-for-service basis. There was, in short, no or little demand-side or supply-side cost sharing. Unsurprisingly, moral hazard ensued, exacerbated by the continuous introduction of ever-more-costly medical technology. In the city of Zhenjiang between 1992 and 1995 total medical insurance expenses increased at an annual rate of 33%.[11]

Most of the past and many of the current CMS schemes operated or operate like the old GIS and LIS in that they passively reimburse members' medical bills. If this were to be the model of the NCMS, health care costs in China would be likely to rise quite dramatically. NCMS needs therefore to think carefully about introducing measures to contain costs. What could these be?

Cost Containment – Lessons from the Urban Reforms

As indicated earlier in this Note, urban health insurance in China has recently been through many important reforms. These appear to have had considerable impacts on costs.

In Zhenjiang, for example, a series of reforms were introduced from the mid-1990s onwards. Initially, these involved demand-side cost-sharing only—patients being required to pay more of the cost out of their own pocket—and costs carried on rising at similar rates. So, in 1997 supply-side cost sharing was introduced—providers were required to take on more financial risk, by moving away from full-cost reimbursement towards a system where the amount paid is fixed in advance. For example, instead of being paid Fee-For-Service (FFS), a provider might be paid a fixed amount for a given casetype, or a budget based on expected caseload. When supply-side cost sharing was introduced in Zhenjiang, the annual rate of increase of insurance costs was brought down from 33% to 15%, where it has since stayed.[11]

The urban reforms in China involved a mixture of demand-side and supply-side cost sharing, and different cities tried different combinations at different times. Furthermore, different cities tried different approaches to demand-side cost sharing. Two approaches developed in the 1995-98 pilots are often contrasted—the pathway model and the compartmental model (Box 2). Both make use of a Medical Savings Account (MSA) and a Social Pooling Account (SPA), with the employee and employer contributing to the former, and only the employer to the latter. However, the contribution rates vary across schemes as does the use to which each of the accounts is put.[6,12,13] The supply-side cost-sharing approaches also differ between the two models.

Box 2: The Pathway and Compartmental Models of Cost Sharing

The pathway model – Zhenjiang and Jiujiang

When any costs are incurred under this three-tier reimbursement system, payments are first made out of the MSAs funds. After the MSA funds are exhausted, the patient pays an out-of-pocket deductible as the second tier, up to 8-10% of the individual's annual salary (deductibles for retired members are half). After the member has reached his deductible, the third tier payment begins to pay by drawing funds from the SPA.

Before 1997, medical providers in Zhenjiang were paid primarily retrospectively at the patient or service level using various fee schedules that varied with the level and type of provider. In 1997, the retrospective reimbursement approach was changed to a global budget approach. Prospective payment was used to pay for all medical services out of funds in the SPA.

The Compartmental model – Hainan

In this approach the MSA and SPA are service-specific, with the former primarily paying for outpatient services and some small inpatient services not covered by the scheme, and the latter paying mainly for inpatient care and some large outpatient bills. Only those drugs and diseases that are included in official lists are paid by SPA, coupled with a deductible (400 RMB) and decreasing copayment schedules, ranging from 15 percent, 9 percent, 5 percent, and 0 percent. Outpatient care services are paid by funds in MSAs on a fee-for-service basis according to a pre-determined pricing schedule.[14, 15]

The SPA has paid providers primarily through a global budget. A current-year global budget is determined on the basis of the actual total medical expenditures in the previous year, adjusted for changing factors such as price inflation and increased numbers of beneficiaries. The Medical Insurance Bureau generally withholds 10 percent of the total budget upfront in order to monitor and control provider behavior during the year. At the end of the budget year, the Bureau will then determine how much of the withheld amount is returned to the provider according to the performance and quality of services delivered.[16]

What have been the effects of the various cost-sharing measures? And what lessons are there—if any—for the new rural CMS?

The Zhenjiang and Hainan reforms appear to have reduced costs to insurers.[17-19] Part of the reason seems to be that providers' unit costs fell. In part this may have been due to the introduction of drug formularies and restrictions on the use of advanced medical technology.[17] But cost sharing on the supply side seems likely to have played a bigger role. In Hainan hospitals shifting from FFS to global budgets reduced cost per case while hospitals that continued to be paid FFS increased theirs.[20] Hospitals in the first group reduced costs by spending less on expensive drugs and high technology.[21] And in Zhenjian, it was not until supply-side cost sharing was introduced in 1997 that spending by insurers was successfully brought under control.[11]

On top of the reductions on unit costs, there is also evidence that the reforms led to patients substituting outpatient care for inpatient care, with the poor substituting the most.[18,22] The impacts on health outcomes are not known, although it is known that during the period in question there was a reduction in the fraction of people saying they had been told they needed hospital care but didn't seek it.[18,22]

While insurers saw their costs fall as the result of the reforms, out-of-pocket payments by households increased. On the positive side, they increased by the same proportion for everyone, irrespective of their income.[23] The reforms did not, however, eliminate inequity: the poor still pay a higher share of their income toward healthcare than the better off.

There is broad agreement, then, that the urban insurance reforms reduced costs. Some questions remain unanswered, however. For example, the available evidence does not provide a clear picture of the relative merits of the pathway and compartmental models. Despite this, it has been the compartmental model that has proved most popular—only Shenzhen has adopted the pathway model.

NCMS and the Rural-Urban Divide

As in other countries, the urban and rural areas of China are not hermetically-sealed entities. People increasingly migrate from rural to urban areas, and this is likely to become an important engine of economic growth. Migrants from rural areas to cities may find themselves in a health insurance no-man's land—ineligible for urban health insurance because of lack of official residency, and likely to be required by their NCMS to return to their village for treatment or risk having NCMS pay only part of their medical bill if they seek treatment in the city where they are working. If the economic benefits of labor migration are to be fully harnessed, it will be important to ensure that health insurance becomes more portable—that loss of effective health insurance coverage does not become a reason to prevent people moving.

As the boundaries between urban and rural areas becomes increasingly blurred, and as the government strives to reduce rural-urban inequalities, there will be a pressure to reduce the stark divisions between the rural and urban health insurance schemes. The gap in terms of generosity of coverage is stark and unlikely to be explained by cost differences: revenue per beneficiary in the urban scheme is around RMB 400, while the proposed revenue per beneficiary in the NCMS is (a minimum of) 30 RMB.

Narrowing the rural-urban health insurance gap need not necessarily involve a merger of the rural and urban schemes, although in some provinces—periurban Shanghai is an example—this seems to be happening. It could happen through a gradual process of moving towards a more equal sharing of health risks. As in other countries, such as Colombia and The Netherlands, an equalization fund could be set up where individuals make contributions according to their per capita income, and insurers receive payments from the fund according to the risk profile of their members. In the longer-term, as the gaps are reduced, it might make sense to bring all Chinese residents into a single universal scheme, as other countries—including The Philippines, Thailand and Vietnam—have done or are in the process of doing.

Looking Ahead, Learning from the Past

All told, China faces many challenges as it tries to extend cover to the 800 million uninsured Chinese, and to deepen the cover of those who do have it. A brave and historic start has been made with the piloting of the NCMS. And many important reforms have been implemented in the urban scheme. But many challenges still remain, as this Note has shown. The good news is that there is considerable scope for learning—from the urban reforms of the 1990s, from past attempts to resuscitate the CMS, and from abroad.

References

1. Sidel V. New lessons from China: equity and economics in rural healthcare. *American Journal of Public Health* 1993;83: 1665-1666.
2. Cretin S, Duan N, Albert P. Williams J, Gu X, Shi Y. Modeling the effect of insurance on health expenditures in the People's Republic of China. *Health Services Research* 1990;25(4): 667-685.

3. Carrin G, Ron A, Yang H, *et al.* The Reform of the Rural Cooperative Medical System in the People's Republic of China: interim experience in 14 pilot counties. *Social Science & Medicine* 1999;48(7): 961-972.

4. Hsiao W, *et al.*, Rural Mutual Medical Care in China. *The Chinese Health Economics* 2004;Forthcoming.

5. Gao J, Qian J, Tang S, Eriksson B, Blas E. Health equity in transition from planned to market economy in China. *Health Policy and Planning* 2002;17(Suppl.1): 20-29.

6. Wang H, Huang G. Assessing the reform models of China's urban health insurance system. *Chinese Health Policy* 2000: 9-11.

7. Ma X, Zhang L, *et al.*, The current status of urban health insurance reform in China. *Chinese Health Economics* 2001;3: 50-51.

8. Liu Y. Reforming China's urban health insurance system. *Health Policy* 2002;60(2): 133-150.

9. Akin JS, William H. Dow and Peter M. Lance. Did the distribution of health insurance in China continue to grow less equitable in the nineties? Results from a longitudinal survey. *Social Science & Medicine* 2003(in press).

10. Huang M, Sun Y. Current situation, problems and reform measures of labor insurance system. *Zhejiang Social Science* 1994(5): 64-67.

11. Cai L, Wan C, Wang J. Analysis on Proportion of Inpatient Expenses and the Influencing Factors. *Journal of Hospital Statistics* 1999;6(4): 206-209.

12. Shen H, Chen X, al. e. Assessing the performance of integration of medical savings account and social pooling account in Shenzheng. *Chinese Health Service Management* 1999;129: 123-125.

13. Wu R. Try to perfect the system. *China Medical Insurance Research* 2004;1,2: 16-19.

14. Wang F. Some thoughts about the combination of the medical savings account and social pooling account. *Chinese Health Economics* 1998;17(4): 34-36.

15. Wang H. Controlling for the growth of medical expenditures using the combined mechanisms of medical savings account and social pooling account. *Chinese Health Economics* 1999;18(4): 40-42.

16. Luo L. Hainan medical insurance practice and thoughts. China Medical Insurance Association Annual Meeting 1998, Beijing.

17. Yip W, Hsiao W. Medical savings accounts: Lessons from China. *Health Affairs* 1997;16(6): 244-251.

18. Liu G, Cai R, *et al.*, Urban healthcare reform initiative in China: Findings from its pilot experiment in Zhenjiang City. *International Journal of Economic Development* 1999;1(4): 504-525.

19. Zou F. A review of the pilot employee medical insurance system reform. 2002;13(6): 66-72.

20. Yip W, Eggleston K. Provider Payment Reform in China: The Case of Hospital Reimbursement in Hainan Province. *Health Economics* 2001;10(4): 325-339.

21. Yip W, Eggleston K. Addressing government and market failures with payment incentives: Hospital reimbursement reform in Hainan, China. *Social Science & Medicine* 2004;58: 267-277.

22. Liu G, Cai R, al. e. China's urban health insurance experiment in Zhenjiang: Cost and utilization Analyses. In: Hu T, Hsieh C, eds. Economics of Healthcare Reform in Pacific Rim. England: Edward Elgar, 2001: 143-158.

23. Liu G, Zhao Z, *et al.*, China urban health insurance reform: equity in cost sharing. *China Economic Quarterly* 2003;2(2): 435-452.

9

Telemedicine in Rural India

Sanjit Bagchi

Basic healthcare still eludes a majority of rural Indians. Although 70% of Indians live in rural areas, more than 75% of Indian doctors are based in cities. Telemedicine promises to be an effective alternative to reach healthcare services to rural areas—it may turn to be the cheapest as well as the fastest way to bridge the rural-urban health divide.

In a developing country such as India, there is huge inequality in healthcare distribution. Although nearly 75% of Indians live in rural villages, more than 75% of Indian doctors are based in cities [1]. Most of the 620 million rural Indians lack access to basic healthcare facilities [2]. The Indian Government spends just 0.9% of the country's annual gross domestic product on health, and little of this spending reaches remote rural areas [3]. The poor infrastructure of rural health centers makes it impossible to retain doctors in villages, who feel that they become professionally isolated and outdated if stationed in remote areas.

In addition, poor Indian villagers spend most of their out-of-pocket health expenses on travel to the specialty hospitals in the city and for staying in the city along with their escorts [4]. A recent study conducted by the Indian Institute of

Source: PLoS Medicine, Volume 3, Issue 3, March 2006. (www.plosjournal.org).

Public Opinion found that 89% of rural Indian patients have to travel about 8 km to access basic medical treatment, and the rest have to travel even farther [5].

Can Telemedicine Bridge the Divide?

Telemedicine may turn out to be the cheapest, as well as the fastest, way to bridge the rural-urban health divide. Taking into account India's huge strides in the field of information and communication technology, telemedicine could help to bring specialized healthcare to the remotest corners of the country [6,7].

The efficacy of telemedicine has already been shown through the network established by the Indian Space Research Organization (ISRO), which has connected 22 super-specialty hospitals with 78 rural and remote hospitals across the country through its geo-stationary satellites. This network has enabled thousands of patients in remote places such as Jammu and Kashmir, Andaman and Nicobar Islands, the Lakshadweep Islands, and tribal areas of the central and north-eastern regions of India to gain access to consultations with experts in super-specialty medical institutions [8]. ISRO has also provided connectivity for mobile telemedicine units in villages, particularly in the areas of community health and ophthalmology [9].

A Telemedicine Program in Action at the Apollo Gleneagles Hospital, Kolkata, India

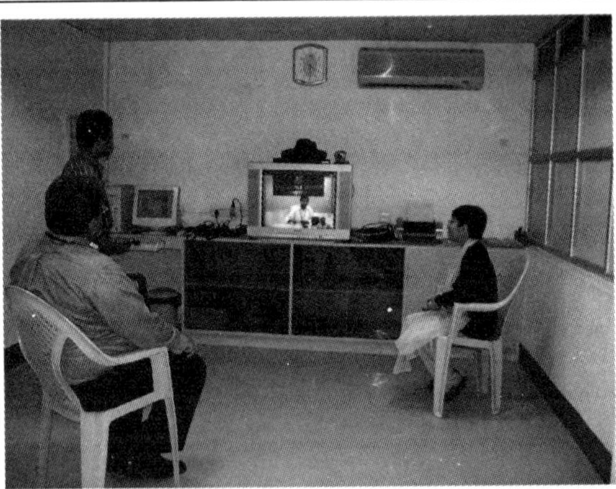

Photo: Nilmoni Debnath/Apollo Gleneagles Hospital.

This encouraging early success in reaching patients—together with recent technological advances in India, such as the proliferation of fiber optic cables, the expanding bandwidth, and the licensing of private Internet service providers—has encouraged ISRO to set up an exclusive satellite, called HealthSAT, to bring telemedicine to the poor on a larger scale. The proposed satellite would not only serve remote areas of India but also those in other poor countries in Asia and Africa. In the Government of India's current budget, INR102.8 billion has been allocated for health [10]. HealthSAT is expected to cost only about 1% of this budget, that is, between INR600 million to INR1 billion. Each receiving terminal (where patients and rural doctors are present for audio-visual conferences) in the villages is expected to cost only about INR0.5 million [11]. This telemedicine service will save some costs, for example the money that patients would have spent on travel and accommodation.

A telemedicine system in a small health centre consists of a personal computer with customized medical software connected to a few medical diagnostic instruments, such as an ECG or X-ray machine or an X-ray scanner for scanning X-ray photos [12]. Through this computer, digitized versions of patients' medical images and diagnostic details (such as X-ray images and blood test reports) are dispatched to specialist doctors through the satellite-based communication link. The information, in turn, is received at the specialist centre where experienced doctors examine the reports, diagnose, interact with the patients (along with local doctors), and suggest appropriate treatment through video-conferencing. The entire system is relatively user-friendly, and only a short period of training is needed for doctors at super-specialty centres and rural health centres to handle the system. And hospital technicians can take care of the operation and maintenance of the equipment.

M N Sathyanarayan, Executive Director of Space Industries Development, and organising secretary of the 2005 International Telemedicine Conference, said: "In the pilot phase of the telemedicine project, ISRO is providing telemedicine equipment as well as making available the required bandwidth on INSAT satellites. The main criteria for funding by ISRO are that the hospitals have to be government-run—state or central—or belong to public sector industries. The hospitals have to provide infrastructure as well as doctors and technicians for operating the system."

"ISRO also provides the equipment and bandwidth to private specialty hospitals and hospitals run by Trusts, if these hospitals provide free service, including specialty consultation to rural hospitals that have been connected in the telemedicine network of ISRO. These hospitals have to provide follow-up treatment to teleconsulted patients at government rates."

In its telemedicine initiative, ISRO intends to connect different types of Indian healthcare centers in a series of phases. L S Sathyamurthy, Programme Director of Telemedicine at ISRO said: "There are 650 district hospitals, 3,000 taluk [subdistrict] hospitals, and more than 23,000 primary health centers in the country. We must aim to connect all these in phases—first the district hospital connected to speciality hospitals in major cities, then the taluk-level hospitals, and finally the primary health centers, so that nobody, irrespective of his location, is deprived of life-saving specialty consultation." When the network grows, it may even include private hospitals as well as hospitals in Asia and Africa. Although the network will initially be used for teleconsultation and postoperative consultation, in the future it may accommodate even telesurgery and telerobotics.

The Impact So Far

Starting with pilot projects in the year 2001, together with a "proof-of-concept" technology demonstration, ISRO has established the facility in nearly 60 remote hospitals, which have been connected with 20 super-specialty city hospitals [13]. A report presented at the Rajya Sabha (the House of States, or Upper House) of the Parliament of India suggested that the initial results of India's telemedicine initiative are encouraging [14]. The report states that several telemedicine projects in India have been successfully interlinked—for example, the Andaman and Nicobar Islands telemedicine project links the G B Pant Hospital at Port Blair with Shri Ramachandra Medical College and Research Institute, Chennai, while in Karnataka, Narayana Hrudayalaya is connected to District Hospital, Chamarajnagar and Vivekananda Memorial Hospital, Saragur.

"There are inevitable difficulties associated with the introduction of new systems and technologies."

Adding to these early reports of successful linkage, there are also reports that telemedicine has helped to save lives in crowded pilgrimage centres and military outposts connected with mobile telemedicine units. For example, the Amrita Telemedicine Programme reports that on 13th January 2003, the programme's first remote telesurgery procedure was performed [15]. The Amrita Emergency Care Unit at Pampa was able to save the life of a pilgrim by a telesurgical procedure using the local telemedicine facility. The cardiothoracic surgeon guided the procedure remotely, and the pediatric cardiologist at Pampa performed the procedure. Mobile telemedicine units were also rushed to the coasts and islands of India after the 2004 tsunami to provide medical consultation and relief to the affected people [16].

There are other indications that the telemedicine initiative may have had a positive impact. ISRO's annual report for 2004-2005 states: "More than 25,000 patients have so far been provided with teleconsultation and treatment. An impact study conducted on a thousand patients has revealed that there is a significant cost saving in the system since the patients avoid expenses towards travel, stay, and for treatment at the hospitals in the cities" [8]. Dr. Devi Shetty, a cardiac surgeon and the Chairman of Narayan Hrudayalaya, a hospital that has served thousands through telemedicine, said: "We have treated 17,400 patients using telemedicine connectivity in various parts of India, mainly from rural India, and [a] few patients from outside India. We use both satellite as well as ISDN connectivity. Now, with the Indian Space Research Organisation, which is our associate in this project giving us the satellite connection free of cost, we have a [larger] game plan of offering healthcare to African and other Asian countries."

The Challenges and Controversies

The telemedicine initiative in India has not been free of challenges and controversies. "There are inevitable difficulties associated with the introduction of new systems and technologies," according to Sathyamurthy. "There are some who needlessly fear that they will lose their jobs. Although the systems are user-friendly, there are others who are affected by the fear of the unknown in handling computers and other equipment. There is a feeling that the initial investment is high and hence financially not viable." In addition, there may be technical hitches, such as low bandwidth and lack of interoperability standards for software.

Discussing HealthSAT, Dr. D Lavanian, an Indian expert in telemedicine affiliated with the Apollo Telemedicine Networking Foundation, Apollo Hospitals, Hyderabad, India, said: "[HealthSAT] is excellent, but some questions remain. Presently HealthSAT connectivity is expected to be given free of charge to certain government entities. This is unsatisfactory as a large percentage of healthcare in India is by private entities." Dr. Lavanian added: "On my requesting to ISRO to open up the same to the private health industry, of course for a fee, I have not received any positive answer. This means that a large percentage of the population of India will be denied healthcare via telemedicine."

These difficulties can probably be surmounted. In the late 1980s, when computers came to India, similar kinds of problems were seen in different parts of the country. That is, people showed technophobia and expressed their fears that computers would cause unemployment and would also be prohibitively expensive. But the country overcame these challenges and fears, and eventually became a superpower in the field of knowledge and information technology [17].

Conclusion

With the aid of HealthSAT, India's telemedicine initiative has the potential to provide specialized healthcare to millions of poor Indians. This potential was well summed up by Dr. Devi Shetty: "In terms of disease management, there is [a] 99% possibility that the person who is unwell does not require [an] operation. If you don't operate you don't need to touch the patient. And if you don't need to touch the patient, you don't need to be there. You can be anywhere, since the decision on healthcare management is based on history and interpretation of images and chemistry... so technically speaking, 99% of healthcare problems can be managed by the doctors staying at a remote place—linked by telemedicine."

(Sanjit Bagchi is a medical practitioner and medical journalist based in Kolkata, India.)

References

1. Agence-France Presse (2005 March 17) India to launch satellite exclusively for telemedicine. Available: *http://servesrilanka.blogspot.com/2005/03/india-to-launch-satellite-exclusively.html.* Accessed 27 January 2006.
2. Krishnakumar A (2003 January 18-31) Healing by wire. Frontline. Available: *http://www.hinduonnet.com/thehindu/thscrip/print.pl?file=20030117007309400.htm&date=fl2001/&prd=fline&*. Accessed 27 January 2006.
3. Rajalakshmi TK (2004 December) India confronts AIDS. Multinational Monitor. Available: *http://multinationalmonitor.org/mm2004/122004/front.html.* Accessed 26 January 2006.

4. Sharma DC (2000) Remote Indian villages to benefit from telemedicine project. Lancet 355: 1529 Available: *http://www.thelancet.com/journals/lancet/article/PIIS0140673605745931/fulltext*. Accessed 22 June 2005. Find this article online.
5. Rao R (2005 May) Taking healthcare to rural areas. i4d. Available: *http://www.i4donline.net/May05/satellitetech.asp*. Accessed 26 January 2006.
6. Ganapathy K (2004) Telemedicine in the Indian context: An overview. Stud Health Technol Inform 104: 178-181. Find this article online.
7. Pal A, Mbarika VW, Cobb-Payton F, Datta P, McCoy S (2005) Telemedicine diffusion in a developing country: The case of India. IEEE Trans Inf Technol Biomed 9: 59-65. Find this article online.
8. Indian Space Research Organization (2005) ISRO Annual Report 2004–2005: Space Applications. Available: *http://www.isro.org/rep2005/SpaceApplications.htm,* Accessed 27 January 2006.
9. *The Hindu* (2005 July 17) IT-based healthcare systems launched. Available: *http://www.hindu.com/2005/07/17/stories/2005071702321000.htm,* Accessed 27 January 2006.
10. *BBC News* (2005 February 28) India unveils anti-poverty budget. Available: *http://news.bbc.co.uk/2/hi/business/4303507.stm.*, Accessed 27 January 2006.
11. *Asian Tribune* (2004 February 12) Satellite to enable telemedicine in rural India. Available: *http://www.asiantribune.com/show_news.php?id=9193,* Accessed 27 January 2006.
12. Wootton R (2001) Recent advances: Telemedicine. BMJ 323: 557–560 Available: *http://bmj.bmjjournals.com/cgi/content/full/323/7312/557,* Accessed 27 January 2006. Find this article online.
13. Indian Space Research Organization (2004 November 29) International telemedicine conference to be held in Bangalore [press release]. Available: *http://www.isro.org/pressrelease/Nov29_2004.htm,* Accessed 27 January 2006.
14. Parliament of India (2002) 108th report of action taken by the Department of Space. Available: *http://rajyasabha.nic.in/book2/reports/science/108threport.htm,* Accessed 27 January 2006.
15. Amritanandamayi Devi SM (2005) Telemedicine at Amrita. Available: *http://www.amritapuri.org/health/aims/telemed.php*, Accessed 27 January 2006.
16. Indian Space Research Organization (2005 January 4) Tsunami disaster: ISRO deploys its resources [press release]. Available: *http://www.isro.org/pressrelease/tsunami.htm,* Accessed 27 January 2006.
17. *New Scientist.com* (2005 February 19) India special: The new knowledge superpower. Available: *http://www.newscientist.com/special/india/mg18524876.800,* Accessed 27 January 2006.

10

Pre-Triage Procedures in Mobile Rural Health Clinics in Ethiopia

PC Stillman and PC Strong

Context: ***Our medical team of 12 people conducted a series of mobile health clinics sponsored by an indigenous relief organization in rural Ethiopia. Coordinating with local health authorities, the purpose of these clinics was to provide acute care medical treatment and public health teaching.***

Issue: ***Initially, we used a 'pre-triage' process that had evolved over a series of previous rural mobile clinic trips. This process involved the lead physician and a nurse-translator moving through the crowd selecting prospective patients based on appearance and responses to simple questions. A significant problem arose when a large crowd of people, desperate to be seen, disrupted the process and jeopardized the safety of our team. We subsequently developed a process that used an introductory session, introducing the team and describing the process of patient selection. We also modified the pre-triage process by involving more people in patient selection. In subsequent clinics, this new process was well***

Source: The International Electronic Journal of Rural and Remote Health, 8: 955 (online), 2008 (http://www.rrh.org.au).

accepted and contributed to increased efficiency and an overall improved community outreach.

Lessons Learned: After experiencing an adverse situation, we developed a system for patient selection that was well accepted and efficient. We found that it was essential to set expectations regarding the purpose of the mobile clinic and the scope of problems that could be treated. This was best done at the outset of the clinic in coordination with local health authorities. In actual patient selection, or pre-triage, we found it advantageous to enlist the participation of the crowd and to send several clinicians among those wishing to be seen for medical care. This new approach to patient selection became an essential element in the success of our mobile health outreach.

Context

The authors were asked to conduct a series of mobile health clinics at the request of an indigenous development organization, Project Mercy, in rural Ethiopia[1,2]. These free clinics were aimed toward, treating acute, non-life-threatening medical problems and providing public health teaching. The overall goal of the clinics was to improve relationships between the communities served and Project Mercy.

The clinics were run from established rural health centers. Administrators at Project Mercy visited each site in advance to arrange for the local health authorities to accommodate the visiting team and to work out logistics and publicity. The team did not specify guidelines for patient selection. At one site local health authorities selected several patients; at others they announced the team's impending arrival but did no patient selection in advance.

The four mobile clinics were set up, and medications made available, chiefly to treat acute disorders. The main acute diagnoses in adults were various respiratory illnesses, gastrointestinal disorders such as gastroesophageal reflux and gastroenteritis, and musculoskeletal complaints. Chronic illnesses included mainly malaria, HIV infection and tuberculosis. In children, malnutrition – including marasmus and kwashiorkor – was a near universal concern, for which we provided a culturally appropriate dietary supplement. The predominant conditions in children were upper respiratory ailments, trachoma, fevers and diarrhea, often superimposed on chronic diseases such as HIV, malaria and asthma. Some less common conditions we encountered were acute mumps, meningitis, lymphatic filariasis, small bowel obstruction, achalasia, and nephrotic syndrome.

Our team included three physicians, a nurse practitioner, four nurses and four support staff. The lead physician was an internist with previous experience working in rural Ethiopia and several prior medical trips. The other physicians were family practitioners, both with extensive experience working in short-term medical missions. The nurse practitioner and each of the registered nurses had prior experience working abroad in various settings. We also worked with six Ethiopian nurses, who were indispensable members of the team, serving as both translators and medical consultants. Each was college educated and worked as registered nurses in the capital, Addis Ababa. They were fluent in English and spoke Amharic and Oromo, the two main languages used by our patients.

All our efforts were coordinated with the local health providers. We stressed to the village elders and the crowd that we were guests of their established health workers and that these providers helped us in all aspects of our visit, including set-up, patient selection, logistics and, importantly, follow-up care. Subsequent communication with our sponsoring organization, Project Mercy, has confirmed that our mobile clinics had a positive impact in each community and served to support the existing infrastructure.

Issue

When we arrived at each site in the morning, the majority of the team set up a triage area, examination rooms and a pharmacy. Simultaneously, the lead physician and a nurse-translator went out into the crowd to start patient selection, a process we called pre-triage. Patients were chosen based on a cursory assessment by the physician and Ethiopian nurse. Several in the crowd were obviously ill, and others were chosen based on the reports of those accompanying the patient.

On the first day at the second mobile clinic, we conducted the pre-triage process without incident. Our lead physician and a nurse-translator started selecting patients to be seen that day. They moved quickly and discretely through the crowd passing out tickets for patients to be seen. People with tickets were sent immediately to the main triage area for intake evaluation. At times, people wishing to be seen would crowd the physician and nurse-translator, but this was easily managed by asking people politely to move back and make way.

On the second day at this same site, the team experienced a major problem that disrupted our ability to provide care. That day, there were twice as many people waiting to be seen by the team. As we prepared to go through the usual pre-triage process, the head nurse at the local clinic suggested that we should move people in groups to make the crowd more manageable. Despite repeated entreaties by the translators and clinic staff to maintain order, the crowd refused to cooperate. People started flooding the area where the physician and nurse-translator were located. Desperate people were begging to be seen, crying and moaning, pulling on the clothes of the team members, some trying to grab the tickets. One woman wrapped herself around the nurse-translator and started kissing her feet.

To disperse the crowd, the physician decided to lead the group outside the gate of the compound. After the entire crowd followed, the team members turned back and flanked the crowd, making it back to the gate, which was then opened briefly for them. It shut before the health educator could get through, trapping her between the gate and the surging crowd. The gate was reopened, which allowed the health educator and 30-40 potential patients back through the gate before it could be closed again.

The team members involved in this incident made a hasty retreat to the back of the compound and began seeing the few patients who had previously been selected and issued tickets. This pre-triage team was significantly shaken by the experience, which they determined not to repeat. We were especially concerned for the safety of team members.

Our Response

When we returned to the Project Mercy compound, we reflected on the experience and redesigned our processes so that we could select patients in a more organized and efficient manner.

We realized that none of the team was well qualified or trained in this cross-cultural pre-triage process. The task fell to the physician who had helped order the medications and was most familiar with our limited formulary.

It was also realized that we had poorly anticipated the size of the crowd, the desperate nature of the people and the sacrifices many had made to get to the clinic. Accordingly, we resolved to use the following approach:

On arrival at the health center, as before, most of the team worked to set up the clinic. Meanwhile, another small group, featuring the group leader, a nurse-translator and the lead physician, would address the crowd to set expectations. During this introductory session (called the talk), we:

- Introduced ourselves and stated our purpose for coming to their village.
  - Explained that the clinic was a result of queries to the local authorities on how best to serve the community.
  - Emphasized that we were working as guests of their established healthcare workers and of Project Mercy.
  - Explained that we were a small team with limitations but would see as many people as possible.
  - Introduced each member of our team.
  - Stressed that the team could not meet the needs of all those assembled.
  - Asked for their cooperation to make the clinic run as smoothly as possible so the greatest number of people could be seen.
- Told the crowd the types of problems we could and could not treat. Specifically, the team:
  - Was not giving vaccinations.
  - Would not treat chronic conditions such as tuberculosis, malaria and AIDS, since the indigenous health system was already set up to address these problems.
  - Was not a surgical team and specifically could not treat cataracts, scarring from trachoma and chronic orthopedic problems.

  - Did not have the supplies to treat chronic fungal infections and certain parasitic diseases.
- Related what problems we had encountered in the past with crowds, and asked for their continued patience and cooperation.
  - Told them that if we felt it was unsafe to proceed, we would have to shut down the clinic and possibly not return to the community.
  - Enlisted the help of the people in the pre-triage process.
  - Asked each of the people waiting to look out for their neighbors and help us identify those who are sickest and in need of evaluation.
  - Reminded them that God would look kindly on those who put the interests of their neighbors ahead of their own.
  - Asked about and accounted for the hardships of travel many of the people had suffered to come to the clinic.

The pre-triage process was also revised. Instead of a single physician and a nurse-translator selecting all the patients, we asked the nurse-translators working with us to participate. The three or four nurses were able to go to different parts of the crowd and could take more time to talk to the patients and their neighbors. This also served to divide the attention of the crowd. Finally, instead of passing out tickets, we had the nurses mark each patient on the hand with a permanent marker.

Each patient with a mark was instructed to go to the triage area. After prior problems with people milling about the clinic, it was decided to cordon off the area, admitting only people with a mark on their hand. Drawing from the experiences of others, we suspended a rope and one of the clinic workers checked for the mark before allowing patients entrance to the clinic[3].

In triage, one of our experienced nurses worked with a nurse-translator to determine the chief complaints. A record was started for each patient, vital signs taken and each patient issued duplicate matching tickets, one to see the physician and another to gain admission to the pharmacy. Each record specified the examination room where the patient would be seen, and in which order.

We found that a specific logistics person was integral to smooth operations. Most of our patients had never seen a physician before and had no idea how to maneuver through our system. The logistics person directed people to correct locations, answered questions and solved problems as they occurred.

Figure 1: One of the Local Community Activists Helping the Team Organize the Crowd Prior to the Pre-Triage Process

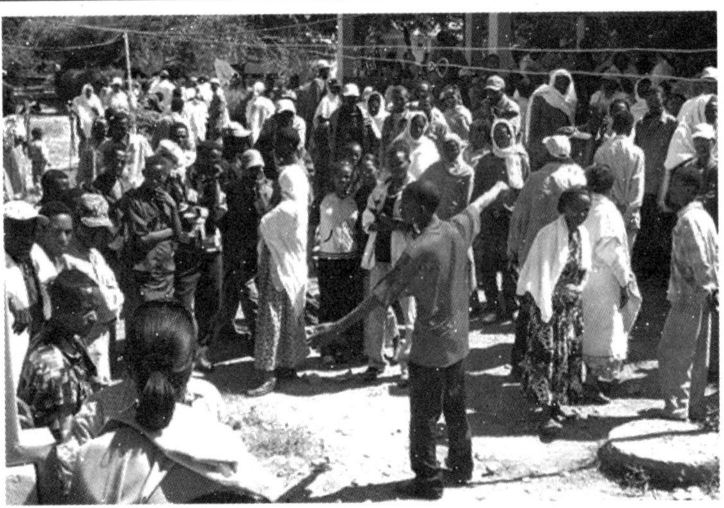

Figure 2: The Team Leader, Chief Physician and One of the Nurse-Translators Communicating with the Crowd in the Talk

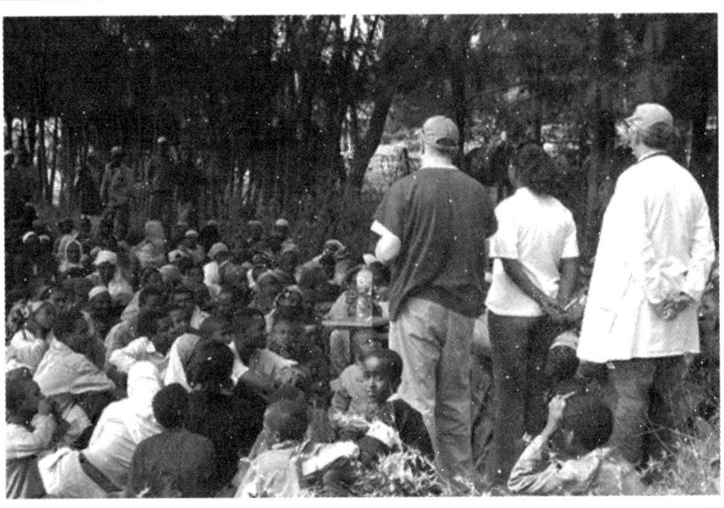

Figure 3: The Physician and Nurse-Translator Going into a Section of the Crowd to Select Patients

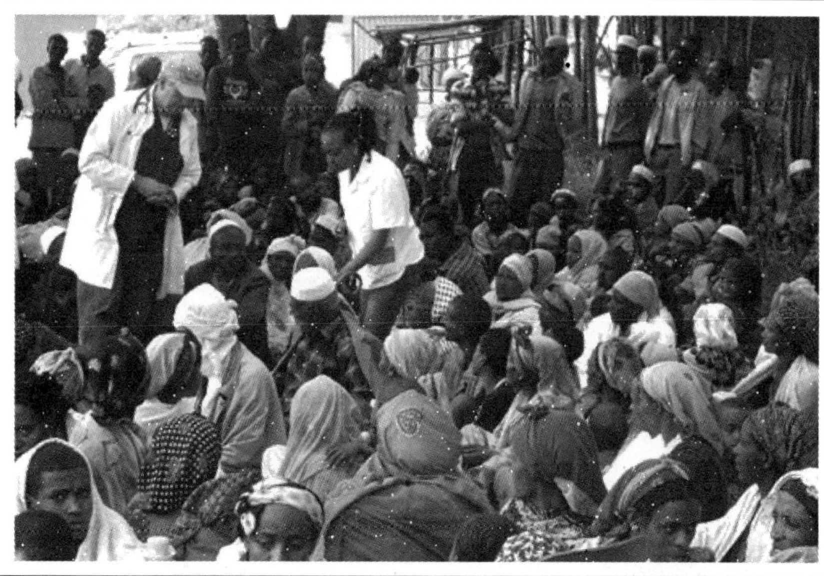

Figure 4: Diagram of the Patient Flow Used in the Rural Mobile Clinics – The New Approach Includes the Introductory Session

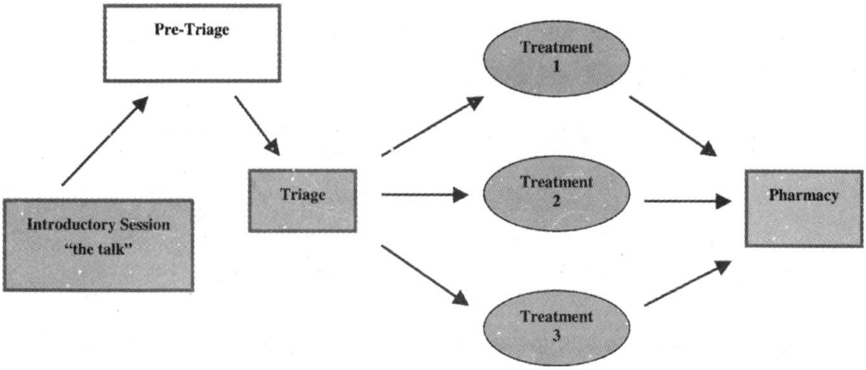

Introductory Session "the talk" → Pre-Triage → Triage → Treatment 1 / Treatment 2 / Treatment 3 → Pharmacy

Result of New Approach

With some trepidation, we returned for a third day at this same clinic. The team leader gave the talk to a crowd of over 200 people. Despite a lack of voice amplification, the crowd was responsive and indicated their understanding and agreement.

Several community leaders were active during the talk, themselves asking questions and keeping the crowd calm.

As the staff from the (enlarged) pre-triage group went through the crowd, the atmosphere was radically different. There were several clear instances of people indicating sicker neighbors or others who had traveled more than a day to be seen. Whenever this occurred, we stopped, pointed this out to the people around us, and spoke a blessing to these members of the community who were proving to be true neighbors. The pre-triage process went smoothly and we found that we were able to see greater numbers of patients as a result.

The same approach was used subsequently at three additional sites over a two-week period without further incident. We also found that the lack of crowd unrest changed how we personally felt about our work in these communities, and we believe this enhanced our work as representatives of Project Mercy.

Lessons Learned

We came to the following conclusions regarding the selection of patients from a large crowd for treatment at rural mobile clinics:

- It is important to correctly set expectations for the group as a whole. This includes communicating the purpose of the clinic, scope of treatment and how the process of choosing patients will be conducted
- Expectation setting is a leadership function. It works best with the involvement of both team leaders and local community leaders. We found that the crowd appreciated being introduced to the team members.
- This can be done with a brief introductory session (the talk) and was best done at the start of the day. This keeps people from the community waiting the least amount of time and facilitates the overall efficiency in conducting the clinic.
- Especially for large groups, it is best if the pre-triage process does not have a single focus but is physically dispersed by distributing pre-triage staff through the crowd.

- A pre-triage approach that actively enlists participation from the crowd, in which they are expected to look out for their neighbors, helps to establish a congenial atmosphere for the selection process.

We found, largely through experience, that the method of patient selection was an essential part of the success of a mobile medical team. It not only established a method through which appropriate patients were chosen, but also set the tone for the entire outreach.

(PC Stillman, Fidere Anesthesia Consultants Inc, Mountain View, CA, USA.

PC Strong, Palo Alto Foundation Medical Group, Camino Region, Mountain View, CA, USA).

References

1. Wikipedia. *Project Mercy.* (Online) 2006. Available: *http://en.wikipedia.org/wiki/Project_Mercy* Accessed 19 July, 2008).
2. Project Mercy. *Homepage.* (Online) 2006. Available: *http://www.projectmercy.org* (Accessed 19 July, 2008).
3. Kuhn W, Kuhn SC, Gross H, Benesh S (Eds). *Global Medical Missions: Preparation, Procedure and Practice.* Enumclaw, WA: Winepress, 2007.

How to Take HIV Antiretroviral Medications on Time without a Watch in Rural Uganda

– Marissa Maier, Mwebesa Bwana, Nneka Emenyonu, Larry Pepper and David R Bangsberg

Castro has advocated that adherence to HIV antiretroviral therapy should be understood within a patient's clinical and social context [1]. Over 90% of worldwide HIV infection occurs in resource-limited settings [2]. Some have suggested that individuals living in extreme poverty may have difficulties with adherence to medication [3], including Andrew Natisios, who said Africans "don't know what Western time is" [4]. While recent reports suggest that adherence to HIV antiretroviral therapy in resource-limited settings may be as good as or better than resource-rich settings [5-7], the question remains: how do people take medications on time without a watch?

Patient with his Radio

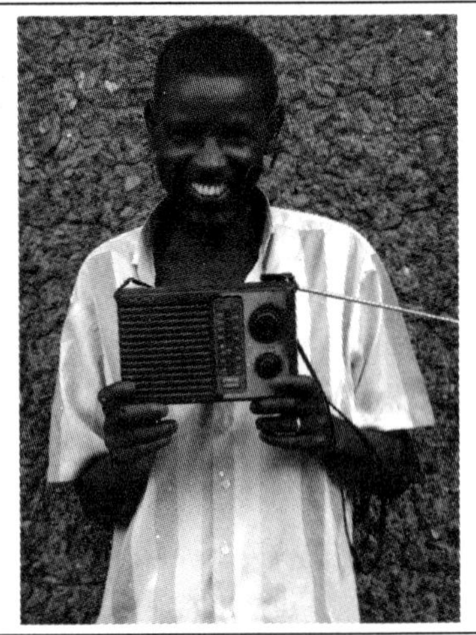

DOI: 10.1371/journal.pmed.0030161.g002

In rural western Uganda, there is, for example, a 40-year-old man who is HIV-positive, has no education, and works as a farmer. He lives with his brother, sister-in-law, and three nieces in a three-room, mud-walled house without electricity.

He owns a lantern, a bed, a sofa, a bike, and a radio, but does not own a watch. He was diagnosed with HIV in April 2005 and started generic D4T/3TC/NVP (Triomune) four months after developing disseminated herpes zoster and Kaposi sarcoma with a CD4 count of 151. His adherence was measured with an electronic medication monitor that records a date-time stamp in flash memory each time the pill container is opened. Over the 89 days of monitored treatment, he had 98.9% adherence by electronic monitor and took 90% of prescribed doses within ten minutes of 7:20 a.m. and within 17 minutes of 7:20 p.m. When asked how he knew when to take his dose, he said that he knows it is time to take his medications by "listening to Radio West's 'News and Announcements' every morning and evening."

Electronic Medication Monitor Adherence Record of Time of Bottle Openings for Morning and Evening Doses

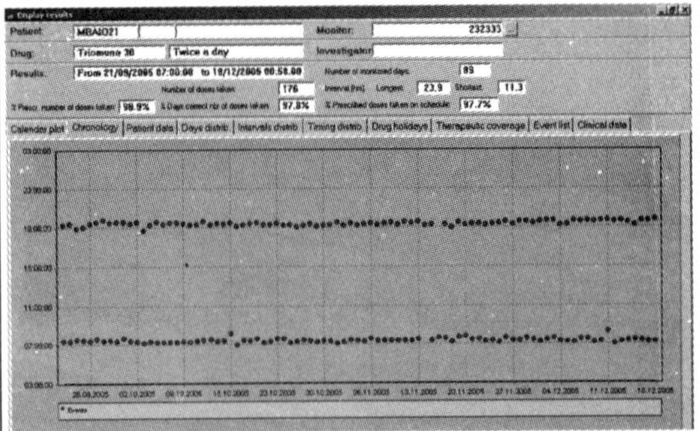

DOI: 10.1371/journal.pmed.0030161.g001

While population levels of adherence will likely drop as treatment access expands and people begin to experience toxicities of long-term therapy, he is an example of how patients can have precise, if not perfect, adherence with creative solutions in a resource-limited setting.

(Marissa Maier, Nneka Emenyonu, David R Bangsberg (db@epi-center.ucsf.edu), University of California San Francisco, San Francisco, California, United States of America

Mwebesa Bwana, Larry Pepper, Mbarara University of Science and Technology, Mbarara, Uganda).

Contd...

Contd...

References

1. Castro A (2005) Adherence to antiretroviral therapy: Merging the clinical and social course of AIDS. PLoS Med 2: e338. DOI: 10.1371/journal.pmed.0020338
2. Russell S (2001 June 8) AIDS activists in uproar over official's remarks on Africa. San Francisco Chronicle; Sect A: 5. Available: *http:..www.sfgate.com/cgi-bin/article.cgi?f=/c/a/2001/06/08/MN164875.DTL*. Accessed 7 February 2006.
3. Stevens W, Kaye S, Corrah T (2004) Antiretroviral therapy in Africa. BMJ 328: 280-282.
4. Joint United Nations Programme on HIV/AIDS [UNAIDS] (2004) Report on the global AIDS epidemic: Executive summary. Geneva: UNAIDS. Available: *http:..www.unaids.org/bangkok2004/GAR2004_html/ExecSummary_en/ExecSumm_00_en.htm*. Accessed 7 February 2006.
5. Oyugi JH, Byakika-Tusiime J, Charlebois ED, Kityo C, Mugerwa R, *et al.* (2004) Multiple validated measures of adherence indicate high levels of adherence to generic HIV antiretroviral therapy in a resource-limited setting. J Acquir Immune De. c Syndr 36: 1100-1102.
6. Orrell C, Bangsberg D, Badri M, Wood R (2003) Adherence is not a barrier to delivery of HIV antiretroviral therapy in resource-poor countries. AIDS 17: 1369-1375.
7. Laurent C, Kouanfack C, Koulla-Shiro S, Nkoue N, Bourgeois A, *et al.* (2004) Effectiveness and safety of a generic fixed-dose combination of nevirapine, stavudine, and lamivudine in HIV-1-infected adults in Cameroon: Open-label multicentre trial. Lancet 364: 29-34.

11

Rural Community Well-Being
The Perspectives of Health Care Managers in Southwestern Manitoba, Canada

Doug Ramsey and Kenneth Beesley

Health care issues in rural areas are dominating the public policy agendas throughout the western world. The issues are many and varied. Canada is no different in this regard, as there are many rural areas with concerns about health care delivery in the face of declining populations. With 80 percent of Canadians living in urban, making the case for designating health care resources in areas with declining populations becomes more difficult. The purpose of this paper is to investigate how health care managers perceive rural community well-being, including indicators of well-being and determinants of well-being. The paper begins with an overview of the literature that places the context of this research in three areas. First, the literature on social capital is reviewed as in recent years both the social and medical sciences have been adopting it for analyzing community health. Second, the determinants of health literature is reviewed as the paper is concerned with the

Source: Journal of Rural and Community Development, Vol. 2, No. 1, 2006 (www.jrcd.ca).

factors (determinants) that affect rural community well-being. Third, an overview of the definitions and models of health and well-being is provided to establish the context for measuring rural community well-being. A model is then applied through a survey of the twenty health care managers responsible for the operations of the 44 health care and seniors' centres located within the Assiniboine Regional Health Authority in southwestern Manitoba. The model also proves useful in identifying determinants of health as well as assessing the role of social capacity in fostering rural community well-being.

1. Introduction

Health care issues in rural areas are dominating the public policy agendas throughout the western world. The issues are many and varied, including distance fiscal restraint, an aging population, rural depopulation, and improved diagnostics (Cloutier-Fisher and Joseph 2000; Kearns and Joseph 1995; Joseph and Hallman 1998; Rosenberg and Moore 1997). Canada is no different in this regard, as there are many rural areas with concerns about health care delivery in the face of declining populations. Within rural areas there are specific demographic challenges, including aging (Pampalon, Martinez and Hamel 2005; Joseph and Chalmers 1995), agricultural (Tay *et al.*, 2004; Stiernstrom *et al.*, 1998), and Aboriginal (Newbould 1998) populations. With 80 percent of Canadians living in urban centres (Statistics Canada 2003), making the case for designating health care resources in areas with declining populations becomes more difficult. Certainly, many parts of rural Canada are facing declining populations (Semple 1981; Millward 2005). Higgs (1999) concluded that more research was needed to better understand the determinants of health and health status in rural areas. Following from this and consistent with other literature work in this area (e.g., Bushy, 2002; MacLeod, Browne, and Leipert 1998; Elliott-Schmidt and Strong 1997; Fuller *et al.*, 2004), this paper argues that it is important to better understand how the people delivering services in rural communities perceive health and well-being. The purpose of this paper is to investigate how health care managers perceive rural community well-being, including indicators of well-being and determinants of well-being.

The paper begins with an overview of the literature that places the context of this research in three areas. First, the literature on social capital is reviewed as in recent years both the social and medical sciences have been adopting it for analyzing community health. Second, the determinants of health literature is reviewed as the paper is concerned with the factors (determinants) that affect rural community well-being. Third, an overview of the definitions and models of health and well-being is provided to establish the context for measuring rural community well-being. In doing so, this paper adopts the four-dimensional model of rural community well-being developed by Ramsey and Smit (2002), as it focuses attention on social well-being, economic well-being, physical health and psychological health. This model is applied through a survey of the twenty health care managers responsible for the operations of the 44 health care and seniors' centres located within the Assiniboine Regional Health Authority in southwestern Manitoba. The model also proves useful in identifying determinants of health as well as assessing the role of social capacity in fostering rural community well-being. The research builds upon the work of Annis, Racher and Beattie (2002; 2005) who established a guidebook of health and well-being indicators for rural communities in Manitoba to utilize in assessing their health status.

2. Scholarly Context

The definitions of rural are many and varied (Hillery 1955; Rourke 1998). Most definitions recognize either or both of the spatial and thematic aspect of rural and community (Ramsey, Everitt and Annis 2002). Rural community has been defined based on forms of association (Haigh and Murri 1990), income sources (Flora and Flora 1988), and a combination of place, locality, and interaction (Cloke 1994). Rural can also be specified or defined based on health care service delivery. For example, Humphreys (1998) and Leduc (1997), developed rurality indices in order to better plan and allocate resources for health care delivery. Others have focused on the issue of distance in providing health care services to people living in rural areas (Joseph and Hallman 1998; Hallman and Joseph 1999; Clarke and Miller 1990). While debates about how to define rural and community have taken place in the literature (e.g., Hoggart 1990; Halfacree

1993; Ryan-Nicholls and Racher 2004), for the purposes of this paper, the definition of rural and small town developed by Statistics Canada is adopted. This definition states that those people living outside the main commuting zone of Large Urban Centres (LUC) of 10,000 or more people are considered to be rural and small town (Statistics Canada 2003). This definition is relevant for two reasons. First, policy in Canada, including health policy, is developed largely based on Statistics Canada data collection and research. Second, the study area of interest in Manitoba meets this definition, with the City of Brandon (49,000 in 2001) being the only LUC in southwestern Manitoba.

The rural condition, or the state of rural, has also been expressed in the literature a number of ways including: quality of life (Michalos *et al.*, 2001), health (Higgs 1999; Leduc 1997), health promotion (Raphael *et al.*, 1999) sustainability (Beesley 1994; Gauthier and Weiss 2005), social capital (Reimer 2002; Diaz and Nelson 2005), determinants of health (Hartley 2004) and well-being (Ramsey and Smit 2002). These are not mutually exclusive terms or approaches as quality of life could be considered a measure of health and well-being and vice versa. Similarly, sustainability has been viewed as the temporal success of measures of quality of life, health, and well-being (Ramsey and Smit 2002). In establishing the context for the research reported on in this paper, three specific areas of the literature were drawn upon: social capital, determinants of health, and well-being. The literature on each is extensive, thus this paper focuses on the similarities inherent to each. Together, the scholarly context provides the framework and justification for obtaining the views of health care professionals (social capital) to identify both indicators of well-being as well as factors affecting well-being (determinants of health).

2.1 Social Capital

In recent years, articulations of social capacity, capital, and cohesion have been submitted as contexts for assessing rural change and condition (e.g., Putnam 1995, 2000; Edmondson 2003; Gauthier and Diaz 2005). Reimer (2002), for example, suggests a model that integrates capacity, capital and cohesion as dimensions for better understanding changes in the rural economy. Social capital and cohesion have also been offered as attributes and indicators of community sustainability (Gauthier and Weiss 2005). Similarly, social capital has been suggested as a measure of what communities and regions have in place to address a particular issue (Gauthier and Diaz 2005). The actions of the resources and the people can be viewed as measures of capacity for a community to respond to changes in health care service provision. A community that is successful in maintaining or enhancing service delivery under constraints and change would be viewed as cohesive.

Social capital has recently been seen as an attribute of health. Pollack and von dem Knesebeck (2004), for example, examine social capital and health of elderly populations in the United States and Germany. The role of social relations in fostering health and well-being has also been addressed in varying ways including placing social capital within the neo-liberal context in which health care services are provided (Edmondson 2003; Talbot and Walker 2007) and examining the relationship between social capital and health, with particular interest in the implications of both on public health and epidemiology (Lomas 1998). Health Canada (2006, 1) recently adopted social capital in identifying "social determinants of health". Citing health as a service example, Rose (2000, 1422) defines social capital as "the stock of networks that are used to produce goods and services in society". This paper draws upon these perspectives of social capital in recognizing that social relations and networks that influence health and well-being. Further, relations and networks are taken to include health care services that are delivered in communities.

2.2 Determinants of Health

The notion of determinants of health is more literal than social capital, that it simply articulates the underlying factors affecting health. What the factors are, however, varies in the literature. Determinants of health have been established for particular segments of the population, including the elderly (Craig 1994) and youth (Rueden-Sieberer, Rajmil and Bisegger 2006), for specific aspects of health (Frankish *et al.*, 2007), and for health service utilization (Muburu, Smith and Sharpe 1978). Kosteniuk and Dickinson (2003) go further by establishing two categories of determinants (primary and secondary) based on social gradients. More important to this work are the frameworks that have been established by the public sector in Canada. As such, for the purposes of this paper, determinants of health will be referred to generally as those factors, either external or internal to the rural community that affect the health and well-being of the rural community.

Several frameworks of determinants of health have been developed by academics and policy makers (e.g., Frankish *et al.*, 2007). Health and Welfare Canada (now Health Canada) view the social and economic dimensions of well-being as determinants of individual health (H.W.C. 1992). In developing a model of health promotion, Hamilton and Bhatti (1996), for example, describe nine determinants of health: income and social status; social support networks; education; working conditions; physical environments; biology and genetics; personal health practices and coping skills; healthy child development; and health services. Social capital is inferred in the networks and services determinants. Hancock, Labonte and Edwards (1999) adapted a somewhat different approach in their identification of six general categories of determinants of health in their model of population health for community-level measurement: sustainable ecosystems; environmental viability; livability of built environments; community conviviality, social equity, and; economic adequacy. More recently, the federal Public Health Agency of Canada (P.H.A.C. 2003) resulted in the identification of twelve key determinants of health: income and social status; social support networks; education and literacy; employment and working conditions; social environments; physical environments; personal health practices and coping skills; healthy child development; biology and genetic endowment; health services; gender and culture.

Based on a research project that brought rural citizens together throughout southwestern Manitoba between 2000 and 2002, a research consortium from Brandon University developed a health determinants' framework, within which indicators were identified for measuring community health and well-being. Illustrated in Figure 1, the framework included ten dimensions, including: education, economics, safety and security, health and social services, environment, community infrastructure, community processes, recreation, culture, and leisure, social support networks, and population and demographics. From this a guidebook was developed (Annis, Racher and Beattie 2002, 2005) was developed for communities to assess their health and well-being.

2.3 Health and Well-being

A commonly referred to definition of health (e.g., H.W.C. 1992, 6) comes from the World Health Organization: "a state of complete physical, mental and social well-being and not merely the absence of disease or infirmity". Building upon

Figure 1: Determinants of Rural Health

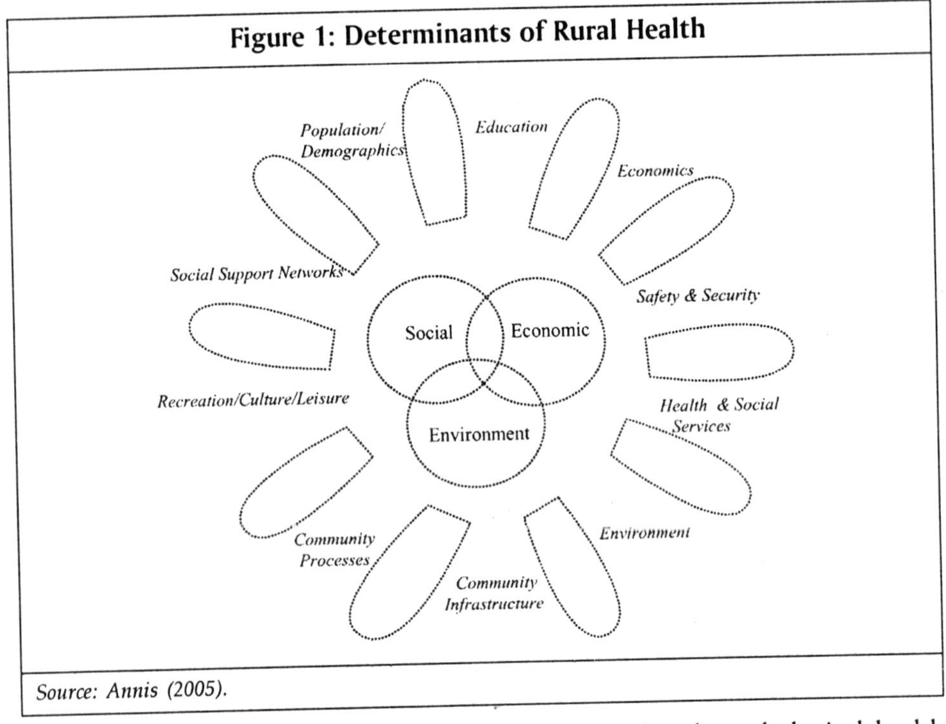

Source: Annis (2005).

this definition, health can be seen to include physical and psychological health as well as social and economic well-being (Wan, Gill and Lewis 1982; Ramsey and Smit 2002; Etches *et al.* 2006). Similar to the literature defining determinants of health, approaches to identifying appropriate indicators of health and well-being are many and varied by both governments (H.W.C. 1992; Begin 1993; C.H.P.W.G. 1994) and academics (Lomas 1998; Pong, Pitblado, and Irvine 2002; Robine 2003; Rueden-Sieberer, Rajmil, and Bisegger 2006). Most relevant to this research, however, is that which the Government of Manitoba recognizes. Based on a collaborative effort by the provincial, territorial and federal governments of Canada in 2000, the Government of Manitoba identified 85 indicators of health that were placed into three general categories and 18 sub-categories as follows:

1. *Healthy Living* – self-reported health, life expectancy, infant mortality, low birth weight, chronic diseases, and health promotion and disease prevention.
2. *Access to Health Care Services* – health information or advice, primary health care, family doctor, immediate care, routine care, ambulatory care

sensitive conditions, wait times for elective diagnostic services, and prescription drug expenditures.

3. *Patient Satisfaction and Quality of Care Received* – telehealth services, community-based care, physician care, and hospital care. (Manitoba Department of Health 2004, 5).

While published after the fieldwork, the framework is relevant to this work given its focus on indicators of both health and health care services.

Modeling well-being and health is not a new endeavour, in fact a range of multidimensional models have been described in the literature. At the scale of the individual and within an elderly health promotion context, Wan *et al.* (1982) describe three overlapping dimensions of human well-being: physical, mental, and social. In a community health context, a parliamentary study for the Government of Australia identified the same three dimensions, albeit with different measurable indicators (P.C.A. 1977). A United States Department of Agriculture study examining how to best target aid to 'distressed rural areas' identified economic, social, and fiscal dimensions and indicators for measurement (Reeder 1990). In a Canadian context, Everitt and Bessant (1992) examined the health of the rural prairies from a regional planning perspective. In doing so, they surveyed both farmers and business operators to ascertain perspectives of individual and economic health. More recently, Ramsey and Smit (2002) modeled rural community well-being on four dimensions: physical and psychological health, and social and economic well-being. This model also established the impacts that external forces of change have on rural community well-being by analyzing a rural community in southern Ontario. In this paper, the model (Figure 2) developed by Ramsey and Smit (2002) is adopted as it separates social and economic well-being and recognizes the overlapping nature of health and well-being. The model is applied in an empirical investigation of a rural region in southern Manitoba, Canada, the purpose of which was to identify whether the overlapping nature of the dimensions of rural community well-being would be recognized by health care program managers responsible for the delivery of health care in rural areas. The work builds upon that begun by the rural health research group at Brandon University discussed earlier (Annis, Racher and Beattie 2002, 2005; Annis 2005). The intent of the fieldwork was to establish a more

Figure 2: Model of Changes in Rural Community Well-being

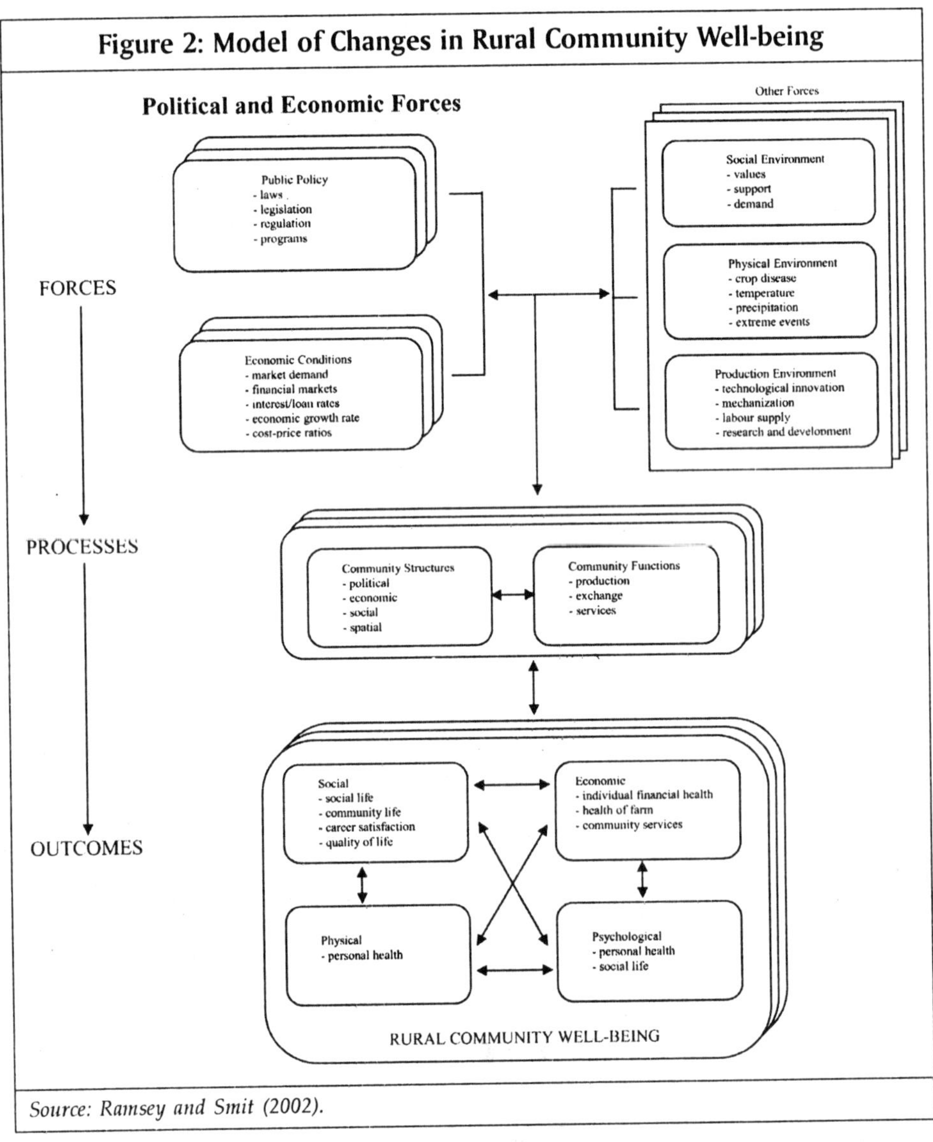

Source: Ramsey and Smit (2002).

comprehensive framework for assessing the importance of changes in one dimension of well-being on others. For example, how do health care program managers perceive change in economic well-being as an impact on social well-being and physical and psychological health? This was explored by having respondents identify both indicators of rural community well-being and the forces that affect rural community well-being.

3. Study Area and Research Methods

3.1 Study Area

According to Statistics Canada (2003), the 2001 population of the Province of Manitoba was approximately 1.17 million people with two-thirds of this total living in the capital city of Winnipeg (Figure 3). The City of Brandon, the second largest city in the Province with a population of approximately 40,000 people, serves as the primary service centre for southwestern Manitoba as well as southeastern Saskatchewan. In addition to having a small university, community college, manufacturing and retail services, Brandon also has a full-service hospital and a number of health care clinics. The rural surroundings of Brandon are served by twenty health care facilities located in smaller communities. Health care delivery in the Province of Manitoba is managed through Regional Health Authorities (RHAs). Southwestern Manitoba (Figure 3) is served by two such authorities, the Brandon RHA (BRHA) and the Assiniboine RHA (ARHA). The BRHA is urban; the ARHA is rural. Thus, the focus is on the latter.

Figure 3: Location of Assiniboine Regional Health Authority in Manitoba

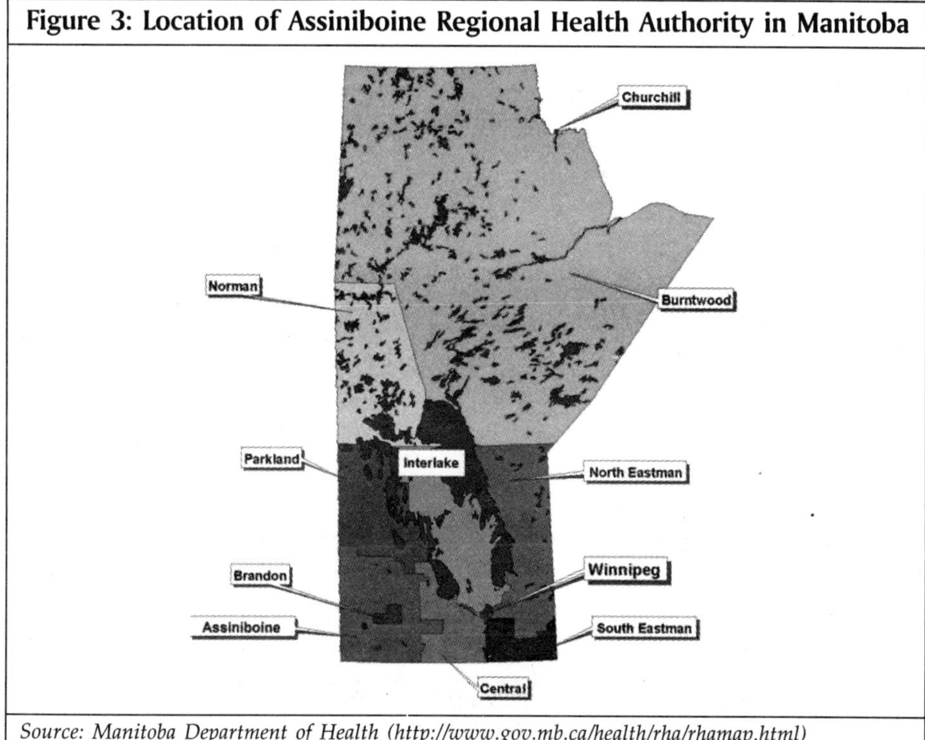

Source: Manitoba Department of Health (http://www.gov.mb.ca/health/rha/rhamap.html)

Table 1 lists the 24 communities within the ARHA, with populations ranging from 304 to 3,325. The communities in the ARHA were classified based on the Canadian Census classifications of Town, Village, and Rural Municipality (RM). For the latter, the three communities listed in Table 1 (Reston, Baldur, Sandy Lake)

Table 1: Study Area Communities and Populations, 1996-2001

Municipal Designation	Name	Services*	Population in 1996	Population in 2001	% Change 1996-2001
Town	Neepawa	H, PCH	3301	3325	+0.7
	Virden	H, PCH	3137	3109	-0.9
	Minnedosa	H, PCH	2443	2426	-0.7
	Souris	H, PCH	1613	1683	+4.3
	Russell	H, PCH	1605	1587	-1.1
	Carberry	H, PCH	1493	1513	+1.3
	Boissevain	H, PCH	1544	1495	-3.2
	Rivers	H, PCH, EHU	1117	1119	+0.2
	Melita	H, PCH	1152	1111	-3.6
	Deloraine	H, PCH	1041	1026	-1.4
	Hamiota	H, PCH, EHU	847	858	+1.3
	Shoal Lake	H, PCH	801	801	0.0
	Birtle	H, PCH, EHU	720	715	-0.2
	Rossburn	H, PCH	581	568	-2.2
	Erickson	H, PCH	507	448	-11.6
	Hartney	PCH	462	446	-3.5
Village	Glenboro	H, PCH	663	656	-1.1
	Treherne	H, PCH, EHU	675	644	-4.6
	Wawanesa	H, PCH	485	516	+6.4
	Elkhorn	PCH	514	470	-8.6
	Cartwright	HC	345	304	-11.9
Part of	Reston	HC, PCH	1710	1567	-8.4
RM**	Baldur	H, PCH	1220	1145	-6.1
	Sandy Lake	EHU	894	837	-6.4
	Remaining RMs		43555	41646	-4.4
Total Assiniboine RHA			72425	70015	-3.3

Notes:

* H=Hospital; PCH=Personal Care Home; EHU=Elderly Housing Unit; HC=Health Centre

** Village population included in larger Rural Municipality (RM)

Source: Statistics Canada (Community Profiles) (2001).

are villages with populations too small to be designated in the Census. For illustrative purposes, the populations provided for these three villages (Table 1) are for the RMs in which they are located. The total population of the ARHA declined by just over three percent between 1996 and 2001. While RM populations tend to be declining, several villages and towns are witnessing either stabilized or nominal increases in population. Apart from Wawanesa (+6.4%) and Souris (+4.3%), the increases tend to be smaller. Further, communities with stabilized or increasing populations were largely growing at the expense of their rural surroundings. This is consistent with the overall trend of declining farm numbers on the Canadian prairies (Statistics Canada 2004). Table 1 also lists the facilities for each community, including hospitals, clinics, personal care homes, and elderly housing units that provide health care services. The range of services among hospitals varies substantially. For example, some facilities have emergency and diagnostic services while in others the level of service is related largely to the number of physicians (from none to five), and their particular specialties.

3.2 Research Methods

The research reported in this paper is based on a survey of each of the 20 health care professionals that either managed health care centers or administered specialized programs in the rural health care centres in the ARHA. While a small number by survey standards, these twenty respondents represent all of the health care centre managers in the ARHA. There were no refusals to participate. In addition, several respondents have shared responsibilities across communities. Because of the small numbers, for reasons of confidentiality it is not possible to identify issues that are specific to a particular community. Consequently, only general observations for the ARHA region as a whole are given. The interviews were conducted from February to April 2003. A semi-structured questionnaire format was adopted in order to obtain respondents' knowledge of the particular topics in question (e.g., definitions of rural and community, indicators of rural community well-being, factors affecting rural community well-being, and prospects for the future) (Peterson 2000; Iarossi 2006).

While every effort was made to conduct the interviews face-to-face, inclement weather and scheduling issues necessitated some of the interviews to be conducted by telephone. This is a limitation of the research, as indicated in the literature, could be possible data differences that could result between the telephone and face-to-face administration procedures (Punch 2003). All interviews were tape recorded for later transcription. In order to provide context in the current study, respondents were first asked to define rural and community. Respondents were then asked to define measures for each dimension of rural community well-being based on the model developed by Ramsey and Smit (2001) (Figure 1). Following this, they provided factors affecting the four dimensions of well-being (forces and structural/functional changes in community in Figure 1). To gain a sense of future well-being in the rural communities, respondents were then asked to offer thoughts about the future of their communities for two time points: in five years and in twenty years.

4. Research Results

4.1 Identifying Indicators of Rural Community Well-being

Respondents were asked to identify indicators for measuring well-being based on the four dimensions of the model of rural community well-being (Figure 1). It was expected that most of the responses, as the respondents managed the health care delivery in rural and small town facilities, would be rooted in biomedical measures (e.g., number of heart attacks); however, this was not the case. In total, 88 indicators of rural community well-being were identified, an average of 4.4 per respondent or one per dimension of well-being. Several important findings can be identified (Table 2). In the physical dimension, respondents described both standard biomedical indicators (absence of disease, rates of health problems, cardiovascular/respiratory ailments) as well as indicators of health promotion (safe environment, participation in activities, having adequate food). In addition to the standard, measurable indicators, these identified indicators of physical health relate to social capital (participation in activities) and determinants of health (safe environment). While only three indicator types were identified in the psychological dimension, a similar distinction can be made between standard medical indicators (stress response) and determinants of health promotion (community involvement). This distinction also illustrates the relationship between social capital (community supports) and health (absence of disease) that has been established in the literature (Rose 2000; Edmundson 2003).

Table 2: Indicators of Rural Community Well-being

Dimension	Indicator
Physical (23)	Ability/Participation in Activities (6) Adequate Food (5) Absences of Disease (4) Rates of Health Problems (4) Cardiovascular/Respiratory Ailments (4)
Psychological (18)	Acceptance/being Positive (8) Able to Respond to Stress (5) Community Involvement (5)
Social (27)	Relationships with Friends/Family (15) Participation in Community (7) Community Supports (5)
Economic (20)	Finances (8) Affordable Housing (7) Quality of Attire (5)

Source: Authors' Survey.

With respect to indicators in the social and economic dimensions, most respondents (15 of 20) identified relationships with friends and family as the primary indicator of social well-being. The overlapping nature of the dimensions was also recognized. For example, participation in the community was listed as indicator of social well-being as well as both physical and psychological health. While indicators of economic well-being included personal finances and affordable housing, it was somewhat surprising that other well-referenced indicators (e.g., employment and education) were not identified. Five respondents identified the quality of attire as an indicator of economic well-being, and explained that when people are doing well economically, one of the most obvious indicators is new and high quality clothing. Indicators such as the latter have been identified by others including Tay *et al.* (2004) who found a direct influence of "material deprivation" on health status and classified as material deprivation.

Several indicators illustrate how interrelationships are important not only in the dimensions of rural community well-being, but also to the connections between health and social capital. That is, the health professionals we interviewed believe that rural resident health is strongly influenced by an individual's connections (participation) in the community, the family bonds and community support that they have, and the presence of opportunities to improve one's health (ability to participate in activities). All of these attributes can be considered to be social capital. As noted in the following section, respondents also considered some of these indicators to be factors affecting rural community well-being.

4.2 Factors Affecting Rural Community Well-being

The model of changes in rural community well-being (Figure 2) describes a host of external forces (e.g., policy, economic condition, environment) that result in changes in rural community structure and function. These changes impact rural community well-being. Respondents provided a mixture of factors that could be deemed forces (health promotion, safe physical environment), changes in structure and function (health care service access), as well as indicators of rural community well-being (genetics, diet). These findings are consistent with the academic (e.g., Hamilton and Bhatti 1996) and policy (e.g., P.H.A.C. 2003) literature that argues for the recognition of social relations and networks as determinants of health. The findings also compare to other work examining quality of life, sustainability, and social capital and cohesion. Raphael *et al.* (2001), for example, established a linkage between community structures and well-being through an examination of quality of life in a neighbourhood of Toronto, Canada. Social capital and cohesion have also been described as factors affecting rural community sustainability in Saskatchewan (Diaz and Nelson 2005; Gauthier and Weiss 2005).

In contrast to identifying specific indicators of rural community well-being as described in the previous section, respondents had no difficulty identifying factors affecting rural community well-being. In total, 164 factors were identified, an average of just over eight per respondent or four per dimension of well-being (Table 2). There was also overlap between what was identified as a measure (Table 2) and factor affecting (Table 3) well-being, with examples ranging from community participation to individuals measures or factors (e.g., finances and nutrition). There was also overlap among the four dimensions for example, employment (Table 3) was identified as a factor affecting psychological and economic well-being. Further, while several factors were mentioned more than once, some by a larger number of respondents, the results illustrate a wide range of 'other' factors identified by only one respondent. In fact, across the four dimensions, 32 factors

Table 3: Factors Affecting Rural Community Well-being

Dimension	Factor
Physical (45)	Safe Physical Environment (13) Genetics (4) Healthy Lifestyle Education (4) Ability/use of fitness Centres (4) Nutrition/Diet (4) Economic Situation (3) Lifestyle (3) Smoking By-laws (2) Ability to Cope with Stress (2) Access to Health Care (2) *4 Other factors mentioned once*
Psychological (53)	Employment (6) Spiritual/Emotional Support (5) Coping/Stress Levels (5) Financial Situation (4) Support Systems (4) Environment (3) Education (3) Home/Community Environment (3) Sense of Belonging (2) Health Promotion/Exercise (2) Access to Health Care (2) Sense of Self-Worth (2) Diet (2) *10 Other factors mentioned once*
Social (30)	Access/availability of Activities (6) Finances (4) Social Interaction (3) Where from/background (3) Access to Transportation (2) Opportunities for Interaction (2) *10 other factors mentioned once*
Economic (36)	Employment (8) Education/skills (5) Personal History (4) Finances (3) Affordable Housing/Lifestyle (2) Access to Human Resources (2) Physical Environment (2) Community Activities (2) *8 Other factors mentioned once*

Source: Authors' Survey.

were mentioned only once. Within the physical dimension, most (13 of 20) felt that a safe physical environment was a factor affecting rural community well-being. Of particular note is the focus on health care promotion, such as lifestyle and nutrition, rather than access to health care services. Similarly, within the psychological health dimension, while stress levels (5), spiritual/emotional support (5) and more formal support systems (4) were mentioned several times, so too were employment (6), education (3), environment (3), and diet (2). The linkage to economic well-being was recognized by several respondents through the articulation of employment (5) and financial situation (4) as factors in one's psychological health.

In addition to opportunities and availability of activities and social interaction, financial situation (4) was also viewed as a factor in social well-being. Only three respondents mentioned finances specifically as a factor in economic well-being. However, financial situation was implied in the thirteen respondents that mentioned employment (8) and education (5). Factors affecting economic well-being also related to the social (community activities), psychological (personal history) and physical (physical environment) dimensions of well-being. Scale was also recognized, with factors ranging from the individual (genetics, diet, employment) to the community (smoking by-laws, access to health care, community activities). Overall, these findings suggest that while it may be possible to identify a core set of indicators of rural community well-being, the factors affecting rural community well-being are more complex.

Another way to understand well-being is to assess desired services in the community (Chappel *et al.*, 1996; Janes *et al.*, 2005). Respondents were asked to state their two priorities for new services if given the opportunity and funding. While in essence a crystal ball exercise, this questioning provided the opportunity for respondents to list services that would truly benefit the community. As indicated in Table 4, the results were consistent with other parts of the interviews if only in the fact that there was a broad range of responses. Of the nineteen respondents that provided a 'number one additional service', four respondents stated that health promotion, as articulated in the identified need for fitness facilities, would benefit the community. The other services mentioned by more than one respondent were also outside of the traditional health centre service provision

Table 4: Additional Services Desired by Respondents

Priority	Service
First Additional Service (19)	Fitness Facilities (4) Elderly Services (3) Dental Services (2) Enhance Mental Health Services (2) Tele-health Services More doctor visits Better lab facilities Primary Care Improvements Minor/Outpatient Services Enhanced Health Promotion Teenage/Young Adult Crisis Seminars More Physiotherapist Visits
Second Additional Service (17)	Chemotherapy Services (2) More Specialty Service (2) More Churches Better Support for Young Families Primary Health Care Centre Better Transportation Improved Mental Health Services Enhanced First Response Services Rehabilitation Programs Enhance Disease Prevention Farm Accident Education Enhanced Elderly Services More Doctor Visits Chiropractic More Social Worker Visits

Source: Authors' Survey.

domain (fitness, dental, and mental health). Eight other services were mentioned once and ranged from better medical services and facilities to health promotion. Seventeen respondents listed a second additional service, of which only two services were mentioned more than once (chemotherapy; other specialty).

The remaining thirteen services ranged from the need for more churches and better transportation services to educational programs (farm education) and medical services (more physician visits). There was also some overlap between the number one and two services (e.g., elderly services and health promotion programs).

Together, the services identified by respondents provide a snapshot that seems to indicate that more is needed than more physicians and specific medical services such as X-rays and other diagnostics. The listing of services such as fitness and elderly facilities also illustrate a broader view of rural community well-being. The importance of place is reflected in the broad range of services outside of the health care domain (e.g., need for churches, fitness centers).

4.3 Prospects for the Future

The last two questions to respondents asked for perceptions regarding the future of the communities where they were employed over the next five and twenty years (Table 5). For each time point, the responses illustrate the linkages between sustainability, social capital and rural community well-being. In the next five years, four respondents indicated specific changes in health care services, all declining or reduced. Eleven respondents described population change scenarios, eight of which related to declines and aging. These trends are consistent with the statistical realities facing communities throughout the ARHA (Table 1). Three respondents mentioned of further hog barn construction modeled on Intensive Livestock Operation (ILO). The issue of ILOs is a controversial one in Manitoba and elsewhere and has been articulated in the literature (Novek 2003; Broadway 2006; Ramsey and Everitt 2001).

Table 5: Prospects for the Future

Time Period	Prospect
Next Five Years (19)	Changes in Health Care Services (4) Aging/Fewer Young People (4) Population Declines (4) Population Increases (3) Hog Barns/ILOs (3) New arena (1)
Next Twenty Years (18)	Continued Population Decline (4) Further Loss of Services (3) Nothing Left (3) Fewer Farms/More Corporate Farms (2) Aging Further (2) Population Increase (1) Volunteering Problems (1) Depends on Environmental Issues (1) Depends on Next Generation (1)

Source: Authors' Survey.

The issues range from odour and pollution (negative) to economic and population stabilization or growth (positive). Certainly, communities within the ARHA have been divided on the issue (Ramsey, Everitt and Behm 2005). In fact, there is currently a provincial moratorium on hog barn construction. While, beyond the purpose of this paper, it was viewed as an issue in it.

The prospects for the next twenty years were gloomier. Most respondents mentioned at least one negative issue, such as population decline, loss of services, fewer farms, and an aging population with fewer available volunteers. Perhaps most telling is that three respondents indicated that there would no longer be a community within the next twenty years. Having said this, one respondent from a larger community felt the population would increase. One closing remark regarding the prospects to the future could lie in the comment by one respondent that the status of the community in the next twenty years depends on the generation that takes it there.

The ARHA faces a number of challenges in the next five to twenty years, including recruiting and keeping physicians. These challenges will persist regardless of how small the communities become. In addition, the ARHA has a challenge to contribute to the well-being of the population it serves, not only in providing health care services, but also through positively affecting and reinforcing influences on rural community well-being. Thus, the ARHA can be considered both social capital (the people, services) and a determinant of health (services) that impact rural community well-being.

5. Summary

The trend toward urbanization is a worldwide phenomenon. For those communities facing depopulation, maintaining critical services becomes more difficult. With 80 percent of its population concentrated in urban centres, providing health care coverage to the remaining 20 percent spread across a large expanse has long been of great concern to policy planners and politicians. Leduc (1997) and Rourke (1998) illustrate this case from a health care provision perspective by developing models of degrees of rurality and remoteness as factors in designing health care service delivery formulae.

The populations of rural communities are aging at a greater rate than their urban counterparts due to a number of circumstances, including out-migration of youth, lack of in-migration to rural areas, the general post-war trends of aging and smaller families, as well as the attractiveness of some rural communities for retirees. Aging populations place a greater burden on the health care system and at the same time this system remains important to the individuals in those communities. This paper has illustrated the issues of rural decline, and in doing so recognized that each dimension of rural community well-being is linked to the others. As the structure of agriculture continues to change, maintaining these communities will remain difficult. In response to these issues, the research summarized in this paper provides an illustration of how one can measure the complexities of rural community well-being by paying attention to overlapping dimensions of rural community well-being and what factors (both external and internal to the rural community) have an impact on the well-being of the community. The results of this study illustrate the importance of, for example, the economic and social dimensions of well-being as indicators and factors affecting indicators or well-being. The ARHA is thus an appropriate and relevant example of the issues of both health and place. It is hoped the findings illustrate opportunities for future research in other rural areas regardless of whether they are declining, growing or staying the same. In doing so, we can continue to illustrate the linkages among various concepts and measures that have been highlighted from the literature, including quality of life, sustainability, health, well-being, social capital and the determinants of health.

Acknowledgments

We want to thank David Bruce (Director, Rural and Small Town Programme, Mount Allison University, Sackville, New Brunswick, Canada) for taking on the task of editing and managing the review process for our manuscript. Thanks also go to the four anonymous reviewers for their comments and suggestions. We also want to thank Amanda Campbell for conducting the interviews and the respondents for agreeing to be interviewed.

(Doug Ramsey and Kenneth Beesley, Department of Rural Development Brandon University, Canada. The authors can be reached at Ramsey@brandonu.ca and beesleyk@brandonu.ca respectively.)

References

Annis, R. C. (2005). *Determinants of Health of Rural Populations and Communities Research Project. Final Report 1999-2005.* Social Sciences and Humanities Research Council Grant 828-1999-1029.

Annis, R. C., Racher, F. E., & Beattie, M. (Eds.). (2005). *Rural Community Health and Well-being: A Guide to Action.* Brandon, Manitoba: Rural Development Institute, Brandon University.

Annis, R. C., Racher, F. E., & Beattie, M. (Eds.). (2002). *A Rural Community Guide for Assessing Well-being and Quality of Life.* Brandon, Manitoba: Rural Development Institute, Brandon University.

Beesley, K. B. (1994) *Sustainable Development and the Rural-Urban Fringe: A Review of the Literature.* Winnipeg: University of Winnipeg, Institute of Urban Studies, Issues in Sustainability No. 3.

Begin, M. (1993). *Our Environment Our Health: Healthy Ecosystems, Healthy Communities, Healthy Workplaces.* Review Committee on Goal 3, Premier's Council on Health, Well-being and Social Justice, Toronto.

Berkman, L., & Glass, T. (2000). Social integration, social networks, social support and health. In L. Berkman & I. Kawachi (Eds.) *Social Epidemiology* (137-173). New York: Oxford University Press.

Bouchard, L., Roy, J. F., & van Kemanade, S. (2006). Developing an operational model based on networks. *Health Policy Research Bulletin*, 12:13-15.

Broadway, M. (2006). Pigs on the prairies. *Geographical Review*, 96(1).

Bushy, A. (2002). International perspectives on rural nursing: Australia, Canada, USA, *Australian Journal of Rural Health,* 10: 104-111.

Chappel, N. L., Penning, M. J., Havens, B., Everitt, J., Annis, R. C., Klein, H., & Kyle, B. (1996). Evaluating support services to seniors and partnering in research. *Home Care Provider,* 3 (1,), 30-46.

Clarke, L., & Miller, M. (1990). The character and prospects of rural community health and medical care. In Luloff, A.E. and Swanson L.E. (eds.) *American Rural Communities.* Boulder: Westview Press.

Cloke, P. (1994). Rural community. In Johnston, R.J., Gregory, D. and Smith, D.M. (eds.) *The Dictionary of Human Geography* (Third Edition). Oxford: Basil Blackwell. 537-538.

Cloutier-Fisher, D., & Joseph, A. E. (2000). Long-term care restructuring in rural Ontario: retrieving community service user and provider narratives. *Social Science and Medicine,* 50:1037-1045.

Community Health Profile Working Group (C.H.P.W.P.). (1994). Community Health Profile. Toronto: Ontario Ministry of Health.

Craig, C. (1994). Community determinants of health for rural elderly. *Public Health Nursing*, 11(4): 242-246.

Curtis, S. (2004). *Health and Inequality: Geographical Perspectives*. Thousand Oaks: Sage Publications.

Diaz, P., & Nelson, M. (2005). The changing prairie social landscape of Saskatchewan: the social capital of rural communities. *Prairie Forum*, 30(1):43-54.

Edmundson, R. (2003). Social capital: a strategy for enhancing health? *Social Science and Medicine*, 57:1723-1733.

Elliott-Schmidt, R., & Strong, J. (1997). The concept of well-being in a rural setting: understanding health and illness. *Australian Journal of Rural Health*, 5: 59-63.

Etches, V., Frank, J., Di Ruggiero, E., & Manuel, D. (2006). Measuring population health: a review of indicators. *Annual Review of Public Health*, 27(1): 29-55.

Everitt, J., & Bessant, K. (1992). Regional planning in rural Manitoba: A study of the 'health' of a prairie region. *Applied Geography*, 12(1): 65-79.

Flora, C. B., & Flora, J. L. (1988). Public policy, farm size, and community well-being in farming-dependent counties of the Plains. In Swanson, L.E. (ed.) *Agriculture and Community Change in the US: The Congressional Research Reports*. Boulder: Westview Press. 76-129.

Franke, S. (2006). What is social capital and why is it important to health research and policy. *Health Policy Research Bulletin*, 12: 6-9.

Frankish, C. J., Moulton, G. E., Qantz, D., Carson, A. J., Casebeer, A. L., Eyles, J. D., Labonte, R., & Evoy, B. E. (2007). Addressing the non-medical determinants of health: a survey of Canada's health regions. *Canadian Journal of Public Health – Revue Canadienne de Sante Publique*, 98(1): 41-47.

Fuller, J., Edwards, J., Martinez, L., Edwards, B., & Reid, K. (2004). Collaborations and local networks for rural and remote primary mental health care in South Australia. *Health and Social Care in the Community*,12(1):75-84.

Gauthier, D. A., & Diaz, P. (2005). Rural adaptation and social cohesion for sustainable development of the prairies. *Prairie Forum*, 30(2):iii.

Gauthier, D. A., & Weiss, S. (2005). Assessing performance: indicators, social cohesion and community sustainability. *Prairie Forum*, 30(2):313-328.

Haigh, R. J., & Murri, D. G. (1990). *Survival Strategies in Rural Canada: The Need For New Paradigms*. Rural Economy Staff Paper, Department of Rural Economy, Faculty of Agriculture and Forestry, University of Alberta, Edmonton, Canada.

Halfacree, K. (1993). Locality and social representation: space, discourse, and alternative definitions of rural. *Journal of Rural Studies*, 9:23-37.

Hallman, B. C., & Joseph, A. E. (1999). Getting there: mapping the gendered geography of caregiving to elderly relatives. *Canadian Journal on Aging*, 18:397-414.

Hamilton, N., & Bhatti, T. (1996). *Population Health Promotion: An Integrated Model of Population Health and Health Promotion.* Ottawa: Health Promotion Development Division.

Hancock, T., Labonte, R., Edwards, R. (1999). *Indicators That Count!—Measuring Population Health at the Community Level.* Ottawa: Health Canada.

Hartley, D. (2004). Rural health disparities, population health and rural culture. *American Journal of Public Health*, 94(19): 1675-1678.

Health Canada. (2006). *Health Policy Research.* Ottawa: Minister of Public Works and Government Services Canada. 12.

Health and Welfare Canada (H.W.C.). (1992). *User's Guide to 40 Community Health Indicators.* Ottawa: Ministry of Supply and Services Canada.

Health, Manitoba Department of. (2004). Manitoba's Comparable Health Indicator Report. November 2004. Winnipeg: Government of Manitoba.

Health, Manitoba Department of. (2007). Physician recruitment positions. *http://web4.gov.mb.ca/physician/list.jsp*. Site visited 24-04-07.

Higgs, G. (1999). Investigating trends in rural health outcomes: a research agenda. *Geoforum*, 30(3): 203-221.

Hillery, D. A. (1955). Definitions of community: Areas of agreement. *Rural Sociology*, 20:111-23.

Hoggart, K. (1990). Let's do away with rural. *Journal of Rural Studies*, 6(3):245-257.

Humphreys, J. (1998). Delimiting 'rural': Implications of an agreed 'rurality' index for health care planning and resource allocation. *Australian Journal of Rural Health*, 6:212-216.

Iarossi, G. (2006). *The Power of Survey Design: A User's Guide for Managing Surveys, Interpreting Results and Influencing Respondents.* Washington, D.C.: World Bank.

Janes, R., Arroll, B., Buetow, S., Coster, G., McCormick, R., & Hague, I. Rural New Zealand health professionals' perceived barriers to greater use of the internet for learning. *Rural and Remote Health*, 5 (online)-436:. Available from: *http://www.rrh.org.au*

Joseph, A. E., & Chalmers, A. I. (1995). Growing old in place: A view from rural New Zealand. *Health and Place*, 1(2):79-90.

Joseph, A. E., & Hallman, B. C. (1998). Over the hill and far away: Distance as a barrier to the provision of assistance to elderly relatives. *Social Science and Medicine*, 46(6): 631-639.

Kearns, R., & Joseph, A. E. (1995). Restructuring health and rural communities in New Zealand. *Progress in Human Geography,* 21(1):18-32.

Kosteniuk, J. G., & Dickinson, H. D. (2003). Tracing the social gradient in the health of Canadians: Primary and secondary determinants. *Social Science and Medicine*, 57(2): 263-276.

Leduc, E. (1997). Defining rurality: a general practice rurality index for Canada. *Canadian Journal for Rural Medicine,* 2(3):125-131.

Lomas, J. (1998). Social capital and health: implications for public health and epidemiology. *Social Science and Medicine*, 47: 1181-1188.

MacLeod, M., Browne, A. J. & Leipert, B. (1998). Issues for nurses in rural and remote Canada. *Australian Journal of Rural Health,* 6: 72-78.

Michalos, A. C., Hubley, A. M., Zumbo, B. D., & Hemingway, D. (2001). Health and other aspects of the quality of life of older people. *Social Indicators Research: An International and Interdisciplinary Journal for Quality-of-Life Measurement,* 54: 239-274.

Millward, H. (2005). Rural population change in Nova Scotia, 1991-2001: Bivariate and multivariate analysis of key drivers. *The Canadian Geographer*, 49(2):180-197.

Muburu, F. M., Smith, M. C., & Sharpe, T. R. (1978). Determinants of health services utilization in a rural community in Kenya. *Social Science and Medicine Part A – Medical Sociology*, 12(4a): 211-217.

Newbold, K. B. (1998). Problems in search of solutions: health and Canadian Aboriginals. *Journal of Community Health*, 23(1): 59-73.

Novek, J. (2003). Intensive hog farming in Manitoba: transnational treadmills and local conflicts. *Canadian Review of Sociology and Anthropology*. 40(1):3-26.

Pampalon, R., Martinez, J., & Hamel, D. (2005). Does living in rural areas make a difference for health in Québec? *Health and Place*, 12(4):421-435.

Parliament of the Commonwealth of Australia (P.C.A.). (1977). *Indicators of Community Well-being.* A Report to the Department of Social Security, Parliamentary Paper No.64/1977. Canberra.

Peterson, R. A. (2000). *Constructing Effective Questionnaires*. Thousand Oaks, California: Sage Publications.

Poland, B., Graham, H., Walsh, E., Williams, P., Fell, L., Lum, J. M., Polzer, J., Syed, S., Tobin, S., Kim, G., & Hardy, G. (2005). 'Working at the margins' or 'leading from behind'? A Canadian study of hospital-community collaboration. *Health and Social Care in the Community*, 13(2): 125-135.

Pollack, C. E., & von dem Knesebeck, O. (2004). Social capital and health among the aged: comparisons between the United States and Germany. *Health and Place*, 10(4): 383-391.

Pong, R. W., Pitblado, J. R. & Irvine, A. (2002). A strategy for developing environmental health indicators for rural Canada. *Canadian Journal of Public Health,* 93:152-56.

Presbitero, A. F. (2006). Institutions and geography as sources of economic development. *Journal of International Development,* 18(3): 351-378.

Public Health Agency of Canada (P.C.A.C.). (2003). What Determines Health. *http://www.phac-aspc.gc.ca/ph-sp/phdd/determinants/index.html.* Site visited 24-04-07.

Punch, K. (2003). *Survey Research: The Basics.* Thousand Oaks, California: Sage Publications.

Ramsey, D., & Smit, B. (2002). Rural community well-being: Models and application to changes in the Ontario Tobacco-belt. *Geoforum,* 33(3):367-384.

Ramsey, D. & Everitt, J. (2001). Post-Crow farming in Manitoba: An analysis of the wheat and hog sectors. In R. Epp and D. Whitson (eds.) *Writing off the Rural West: Globalization, Governments, and the Transformation of Rural Life.* University of Alberta Press: Edmonton. 3-20.

Ramsey, D., Annis, R. C., & Everitt, J. (2002). Definitions and boundaries of community: The case of rural health focus group analysis in southwestern Manitoba. *Prairie Perspectives: Geographical Essays,* 5:187-201.

Ramsey, D., Annis, R. C., & Everitt, J. (2003). Rural community in Westman: Theoretical and empirical Considerations. In R. Blake and A. Nurse (eds.) The Trajectories of Rural Life: New Perspectives on Rural Canada. Canadian Plains Research Centre, University of Regina. 1-10.

Ramsey, D., Everitt, J., & Behm, L. (2005). People and hogs: Agricultural restructuring and the contested countryside in agro-Manitoba. In S. Essex (ed.) *Contrasting Ruralities: Changing Rural Economies, Societies and Landscapes.* U.K.:CABI. 48-67.

Raphael, D., Renwick, R., Brown, I., Steinmetz, B., Sehdev, H., & Phillips, S. (2001). Making the links between community structure and individual well-being: Community quality of life in Riverdale, Toronto, Canada. *Health and Place,* 7:179-196.

Raphael, D., Steinmetz, B., Renwick, R., Rootman, I., Brown, I., Sehdev, H., Phillips, S., & Smith, T. (1999). The community quality of life project: A health promotion approach to understanding communities. *Health Promotion International,* 14(3): 197-210.

Reeder, R. J. (1990). *Targeting Aid to Distressed Rural Areas: Indicators of Fiscal and Community Well-being.* Agriculture and Rural Economy Division, Economic Research Service, US Department of Agriculture. Staff Report No. AGES 9067. Washington, D.C.

Reimer, B. (2002). Sample frame for rural Canada: Design and evaluation. *Regional Studies,* 36:845-859.

Robine, J. M. (2003). The relevance of population health indicators. *Journal of Epidemiology and Community Health,* 57(5): 318.

Rose, R. (2000). How much does social capital add to individual health? A survey study of Russians. *Social Science and Medicine*, 51(9): 1421-1435.

Rosenberg, M. W., & Moore, E. G. (1997). The health of Canada's elderly population: Current status and future implications. *Canadian Medical Association Journal*, 157:1025-1032.

Rourke, J. (1998). In search of a definition of 'rural'. *Canadian Journal of Medicine*, 2: 113-115.

Rueden-Sieberer, U., Rajmil, L., & Bisegger, C. (2006). Socioeconomic determinants of health related quality of life in childhood and adolescence: Results from a European Study. *Journal of Epidemiology and Community Health*, 60(2): 130-135.

Ryan-Nicholls, K. D., & Racher, F. (2004). Investigating the health of rural communities: toward framework development. *Rural and Remote Health*, 4(online)-244: 1-10.

Semple, R. K. (1981). A geographical perspective of the prairies: the 1980s. *Manitoba Geographical Studies*, 7:106-123.

Statistics Canada. (2003). *2001 Census: Age and Sex Profile: Canada*. (*www.12statcan.ca/english/census01/Products/Analytic/companion/age/canada.ca*).

Statistics Canada. (2004). *Canadian Agriculture at a Glance*. Agriculture Division, Statistics Canada, Ottawa, Ontario, Canada.

Stiernstrom, E. L., Holmberg, S., Thelin, A., & Svardsudd, K. (1998). Reported health status among farmers and nonfarmers in nine rural districts. *Journal of Occupational and Environmental Medicine*, 40(19): 917-924.

Talbot, L. & Walker, R. (2007). Community perspectives on the impact of policy change on linking social capital in a rural community. *Health and Place*, 13: 482-492.

Tay, J. B., Kellerher, C. C., Hope, A., Barry, M., Gabhainn, S. N., & Sixsmith, J. (2004). Influence of sociodemographic and neighbourhood factors on self rated health and quality of life in rural communities: findings from the Agriproject in the republic of Ireland. *Journal of Epidemiology and Community Health*, 58(11): 904-911.

Van Kemenade, S. (2003). *Social Capital as a Health Determinant – How is it Defined?* Health Policy Research Working Paper Series. Ottawa: Minister of Public Works and Government Services Canada.

Wan, T., Gill Odell, B., & Lewis, D. (1982). *Promoting Well-Being of the Elderly: A Community Diagnosis*. New York: Haworth Press.

Worley, P. S. (2005). Rural and remote communities – Innovation in the midst of adversity. *Rural and Remote Health* 5 (online)- 458: 1-2. Available from: *http://www.rrh.org.au*

12

Health Security for Rural Poor

Study of Community-Based Health Insurance System in India

Sudha Menon

This article highlights the need for health insurance schemes in rural India especially in the context of increasing health expenditure burden over the poor and lack of public healthcare spending. The need for community-based health insurance scheme is analyzed with a case study of Chaitanya-HDFC Chub Insurance scheme successfully implemented in Maharashtra.

Introduction

Developing countries account for 84% of the world's population, and 93% of the worldwide burden of disease. These figures starkly contrast the fact that these very nations account for only 18% of global income, and a meager 11% of global health spending. Furthermore, of the 1.4 trillion Disability-Adjusted Life Years (DALYs) lost annually around the world, the developing world accounts for an overwhelming 93% of this burden, while industrialized nations represent a mere 7% of lost years [Schieber, G and Maeda A: 1999]. DALYs are a measure by

Source: Insurance Chronicle, April 2007.

which international development agencies quantify the burden of disease. In layman's terms, DALYs account for the years of life lost due to the effects of disease that are calculated using a two-thirds mortality and one-third morbidity ratio.

In the developing world, South Asia, which is predominantly represented by India, ranks amongst the lowest in health spending: it is a central problem that hinders India's ability to advance its society. Table 1 illustrates South Asia's global position in health spending.

Table 1: Global Distribution of Health Spending, and Population among Low- and Middle-Income Countries (1994)

	Gross Domestic Product (%)	Health Spending (%)	Population (%)
East Asia and Pacific	24	17	35
Europe and Central Asia	19	18	11
Latin America and Caribbean	35	42	9
Middle East and North Africa	8	9	7
South Asia	9	8	26
Sub-Saharan Africa	5	6	12

Source: The World Bank Health, Nutrition and Population, 1994, Database.

India's Public Healthcare Funding

The healthcare financing situation in India is dire indeed. According to a 2001 report issued by the World Bank, public spending on health in India is less than 1% of India's GDP, poor in comparison with the average distribution of 2.8% in low and middle-income countries [Ahuja: 2004]. Overall, public spending is inadequate to meet the needs of Indian people and is even too deficient to provide the most basic healthcare to the population. Furthermore, the government allocates the bulk of public spending to primary healthcare funds that are spread too thinly to provide effective care [World Bank: 2001].

While the government's inadequate health spending alone contributes significantly to the insufficient healthcare provided to its population, substandard distribution of these funds worsens India's health spending problems. Of the money allocated for public health spending by the government, a disproportionately large amount is spent on salaries and staff logistics, while only a fraction of a percent is spent on actual user fees. Figure 1 illustrates the asymmetrical distribution of public health spending.

Figure 1: India's Limited Public Health Spending is Poorly Distributed

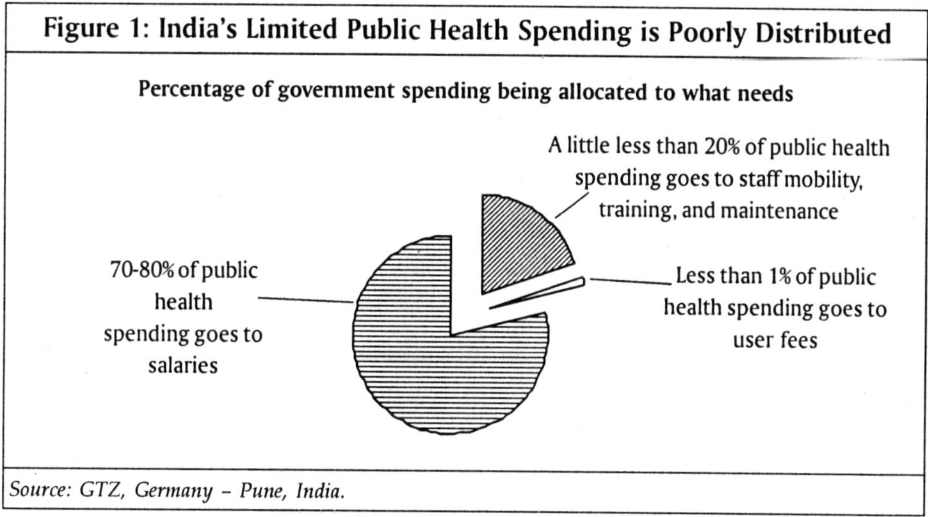

Source: GTZ, Germany – Pune, India.

In addition to the deficient allocation, limited public spending by the government is not, as one may assume, distributed solely among the underprivileged, but is also utilized by affluent sections of the society. In fact, when dealing with curative public services, the wealthier section of Indian society receives almost three rupees of care for every one rupee of care provided to the poorest fifth of the population. Parallel to the difference in monetary allocation of care, there are also large disparities in the distribution of types of services between classes of society. Health spending for the poorer sections of the population focuses greatly on primary healthcare services such as immunizations and other outpatient procedures, whereas inpatient care is less likely to reach poorer populations [World Bank: 2001].

Shortcomings of Public Health Delivery in India

It has been estimated that close to 87% of total health spending in India is private, and of that, 84.6% is out-of-pocket, point-of-service expenditure, lower only to Cambodia, the Democratic Republic of Congo, Georgia, Myanmar, and Sierra Leone [Ahuja: 2004]. Although state facilities exist, the lack of their funding and blatant shortcomings force India's population, even the rural poor, to rely on private providers for their healthcare needs. This is because the poor generally have higher rates of morbidity and are more prone to disease, they are often required to pay more for their healthcare. Therefore, private expenditure leave vulnerable sections of society most affected by these forms of payment [World Bank: 2005].

The current rural health system is organized into three tiers: The first and most basic tier is the sub-center, which provides healthcare for 5,000 people in general areas and for 3,000 people in hilly, tribal, and backward areas. The second tier consists of Primary Health Centers (PHCs), which provide care for 30,000 people in general areas and 20,000 people in hilly, tribal, and backward areas (Figure 2). PHCs are responsible for all ambulatory illness treatment services, routine preventive care practices, outpatient maternity care, as well as public health control measures. Finally, Community Health Centers (CHCs) make up the last of the three tiers providing medicare for 80,000 to 1,20,000 people and specialized services in gynaecology, pediatrics, surgery, and medicine.

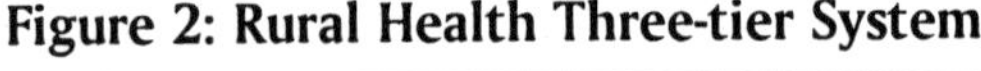

Figure 2: Rural Health Three-tier System

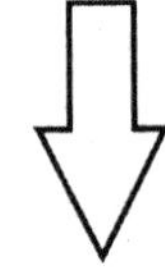

Sub-centers: 3,000 to 5,000 people covered.

Primary Health Centers (PHCs): 20,000 to 30,000 people covered.

Community Health Centers (CHCs): 80,000 to 1,20,000 people covered.

Inspite of this structure in the rural healthcare system, various problems exist. Firstly, the public health system is understaffed and overtaxed resulting in an acute shortage of healthcare workers, leaving posts unfilled and care undelivered. In comparison to staffing norms established for sub-centers, PHCs, and CHCs, current numbers exhibit a shortfall of approximately 28,000 Auxiliary Nurse Midwives (ANMs), 65,000 male multipurpose workers, 21,000 nurse midwives, and 10,000 doctors. Additionally, money is misallocated for rural healthcare as it is primarily spent on salaries, with a minimum percentage used for drugs, supplies, transport of patients, or maintenance.

Studies show that people in rural areas are dissatisfied with the provided services. Reasons for this dissatisfaction are various: PHCs are generally far in distance, forcing people to walk or find some other mode of transportation in order to seek care. Even if people are able to reach the PHC, often the physician is either not present or unavailable to provide treatment. When people finally see a physician, prescriptions written often require people to travel another long distance to obtain medicines.

There is a significant shortage of medicines, as well as a lack of emergency equipment and life-saving drugs. Finally, long waiting hours and unsympathetic staff create additional reasons for rural poor populations dissatisfied with the public health system. Additionally, the rural public health sector lacks any structure for monitoring and quality assurance, resulting in the deliverance of the aforesaid inadequate care [World Bank: 2001].

This widespread dissatisfaction with the public rural system causes rural poor populations to seek private care or go to traditional healers for their health needs. In fact, a health study conducted in 1997 at the Harvard School of Public Health showed that 82% of illness episodes in rural areas went to private practitioners for whom individuals were required to pay out-of-pocket, at the point of service [Berman: 1997].

Private Spending Perpetuates the Poverty Cycle

The trend of out-of-pocket health spending places the burden of health financing on the individual as opposed to the state, often causing poor families to fall below the poverty line. Although, the rural poor are significantly less likely to be hospitalized for an ailment, the frequent occurrence of hospitalization can result in catastrophic financial consequences for a poor family, especially without risk-pooling mechanisms to help families pull through times of illness [Garg: 1998]. Recent studies show that only 10% of India's population is covered under some form of risk-pooling. Hospitalized Indians who are predominantly the non-poor, spent more than 53% of their total annual expenditures on healthcare and close to 40% of those hospitalized borrow money or sell assets to cover health costs. Families that are obliged to borrow money or sell assets to finance their care are, as a result, frequently pushed under the poverty line. Figure 3 demonstrates the percentage of hospitalized Indians who fall below the poverty line due to hospitalization costs.

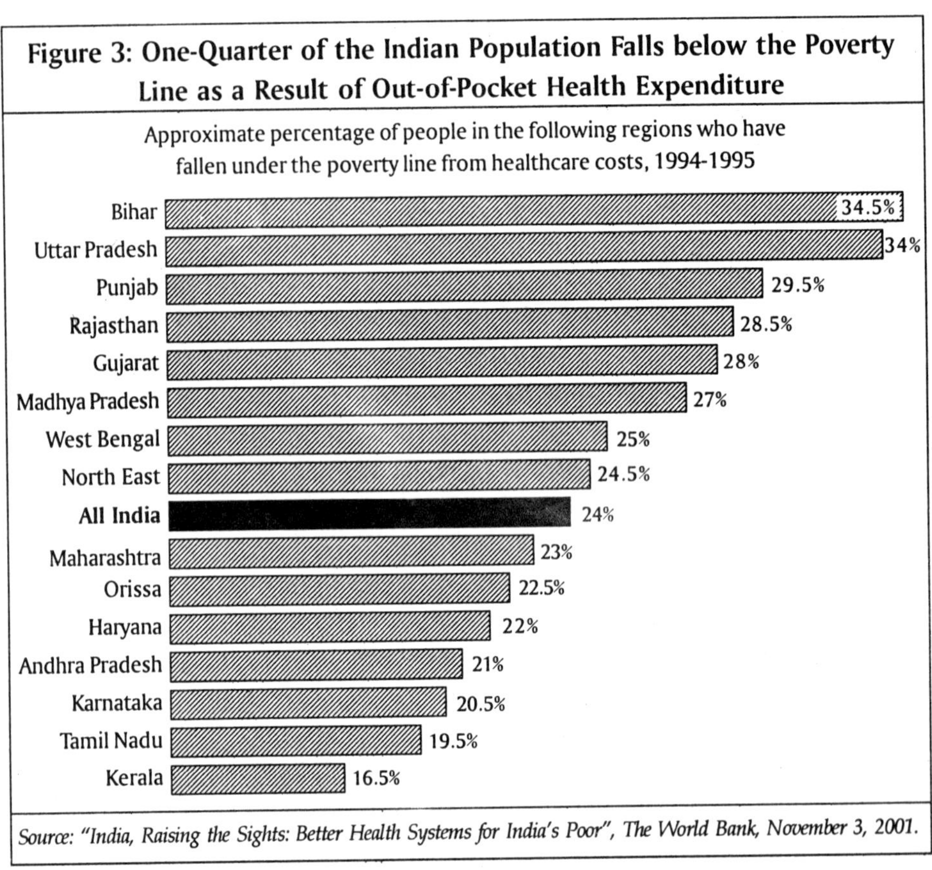

Figure 3: One-Quarter of the Indian Population Falls below the Poverty Line as a Result of Out-of-Pocket Health Expenditure

Source: "India, Raising the Sights: Better Health Systems for India's Poor", The World Bank, November 3, 2001.

Need for Health Financing in India

As the figures demonstrate, for many people living in developing nations, illness represents a permanent threat to their income earning capacity and, therefore, their livelihood. Health insurance (i.e., the practice of risk-pooling) has been progressively more recognized as a tool to finance healthcare provision in the developing world. The high demand for good quality healthcare and the extreme underutilization of existing health services have given rise to the need for community health insurance—an arrangement that may both increase access to healthcare as well as theoretically improve its quality. While alternative forms of healthcare financing have been considered, the option of insurance seems to be promising as it offers the opportunity to pool risk by converting unpredictable healthcare costs into fixed annual premiums.

Community-Based Health Insurance

The typical dialog surrounding health financing cites three main types of insurance as viable options to provide care. First is social health insurance, a practice initiated in several European countries where the working population of society provides health funds for the entire population, working and non-working. Social health insurance utilizes basic socialist principles to hold all sections of society accountable for the good of the community. The next type of insurance model is private health insurance, a structure that generally prevails in capitalist societies. Private insurance favors those who can afford to pay regular premia, i.e., the middle-class and the wealthy. Private insurance, therefore, inherently excludes the poor and only provides benefits to paying members. Finally, the most notable model of health for the rural poor, is Community-Based Health Insurance (CBHI).

Studies conducted in various developing countries, including India, show that CBHI schemes are highly effective in reaching poor populations. According to Friends of Women's World Banking, CBHI is defined as "Any not-for-profit insurance scheme that is aimed primarily at the informal sector and formed on the basis of a collective pooling of health risks, and the members participate in its management." Such schemes frequently function in conjunction with healthcare providers or community organizations, such as local religious institutions, Self-Help Groups (SHGs), or Non-Governmental Organizations (NGOs).

CBHI requires that people make a small contribution (i.e., pay a premium), which is then pooled to provide benefits, such as medical costs, to those within the pool who may need assistance. Unlike social or private health insurance schemes, CBHI is distinct in that it is generally initiated and managed by the community it benefits. This characteristic of CBHI is particularly important as it entails that the features of any specific CBHI scheme are tailored to the local needs of the people (Figure 4).

In fact, specifically in regard to low administrative costs, studies estimate that the average health insurance provider has to spend close to 20% of its premium amount on staff, who are hired to popularize the idea of insurance, collect premia, verify claims, and then ultimately reimburse them. In contrast, such costs can be

Figure 4: CBHI Schemes Tailored to the Community Needs
Communal benefits of CBHI, in no specific order
#1 Community-owned; therefore, supported by a strong will to want it to succeed.
#2 Design agrees with the needs of the community; therefore likely to be more effective in caring for beneficiaries.
#3 Often managed or co-managed by the people, resulting in minimal overhead administrative costs, if at all.
#4 Effective in reducing informational asymmetries.
Sources: "Community Health Insurance in India", Friends of Women's World Banking, India. April 2005; Ahuja, R "Health Insurance for the Poor in India" and Indian Council for Research on International Economic Relations, March 2004.

minimized to a mere 5 to 6% of premium amounts for CBHI schemes, where the community manages or co-manages administrative tasks by itself. Finally, CBHI has been known to make specific efforts to not only improve healthcare access to the rural poor, but also to help fill gaps in levels of knowledge these target communities have regarding basic health information. Therefore, the health insurance schemes serve to improve access to healthcare systems, while also improving healthcare education for these marginalized populations.

CBHI Schemes Take on Various Shapes

To date, there are approximately 30 CBHI schemes across India conservatively covering 3.5 million Indians [World Bank: 2005]. Each of these implemented schemes presents unique characteristics as an inherent feature of their being tailored to the communities they serve. As a result, CBHI schemes have been established using multiple techniques of administration and efficiency practices.

CBHI schemes generally assume one of three main models: The provider model, the insurer model, and the linked model. In the provider model, the NGO acts as both the provider of healthcare as well as the agent collecting premiums and needed funds. Taking a slightly more distant approach, in the insurer model, the NGO, in conjunction with other Community-Based Organizations (CBOs), acts solely as the insurance agency, requiring them to either purchase healthcare services from a network of providers or reimburse CBHI members after having received and paid for care. Lastly, in the linked model, NGOs and CBOs act as intermediaries between the insurance agency, the providers, and the insured members. Figure 5 depicts the variety of roles NGOs can assume.

Figure 5: NGOs Play Different Roles in CBHI

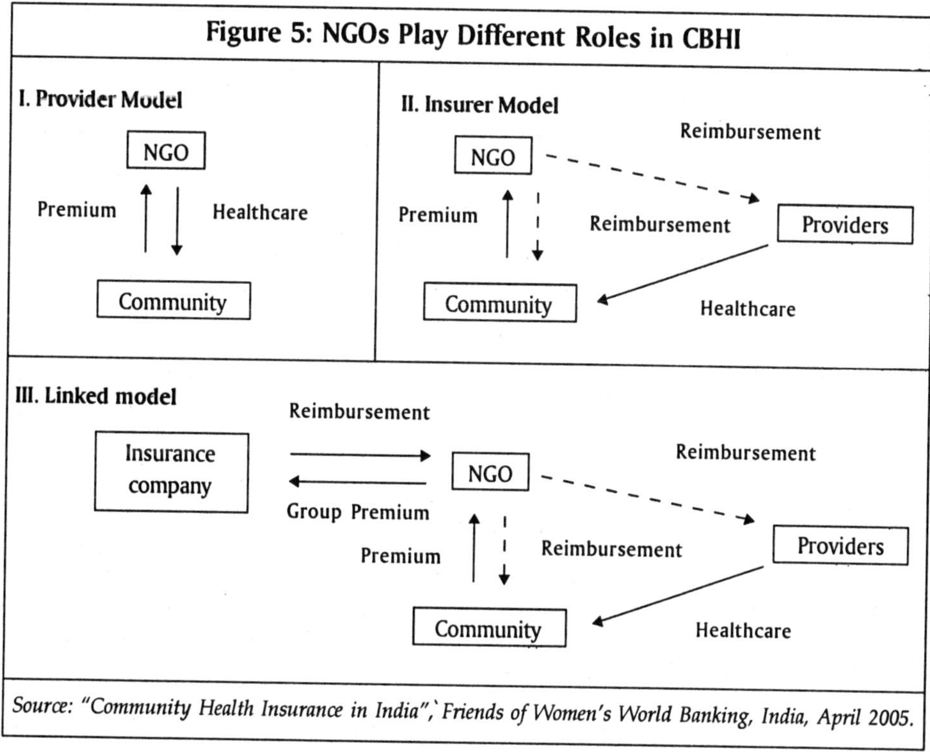

Source: "Community Health Insurance in India", Friends of Women's World Banking, India, April 2005.

Each of these three models carries with it specific characteristics that are often examined through the evaluation of the following parameters: Freedom to suit the local needs, premia, benefit packages, financial risks, quality of care and community involvement. For instance, the provider model allows for maximum flexibility in suiting local needs as the NGO sees fit, while the linked model scheme must function depending on the parameters of the insurance company employed. Similarly for premia, the provider and insurer models usually base their premia on affordability and are set by NGOs and CBOs, whereas insurance companies dictate premia set through the linked model. Benefit packages for linked CBHI schemes are restricted to the insurance provider and almost always have policy limitations and exclusions, while provider and insured schemes are open to include benefits relevant to the people.

When it comes to financial risk, the provider and insurer models carry the maximum risk, while the linked model places the highest financial burden on the insurance company itself. As for the quality of care, theoretically, it should improve with the provider and insurer models because they cater directly to the community. However, with financial constraints, in application, the linked model may actually provide the highest quality of care. Community involvement is almost entirely dependent on each individual scheme and the parameters set by the insurance companies, the healthcare providers, the NGOs and the CBOs.

CBHI Schemes Still Fall Short on Several Fronts

While CBHI models appear to be ideal solutions to the healthcare issues of the rural poor, like all developmental schemes, they also have shortcomings that affect their success. For one, the unique traits of each scheme make it nearly impossible to establish a pan-India CBHI scheme, which creates severe barriers to replicating the plans for future application. Furthermore, CBHI schemes are not financially padded and therefore, highly vulnerable to bankruptcy in the event of a catastrophe. Finally, as a result of their organic nature, such insurance plans tend to lack technical expertise, which may lead to significant impediments in effectiveness and efficiency.

Perhaps the most alarming drawback, however, even despite their focus on affordability and the community, is that CBHI schemes are not able to protect the poorest segments of the community. While this is a failing of almost all types of insurance, it appears most glaring for CBHI schemes that came about as a means to help the ultra-poor population. It is said that unfortunately a large segment of the Indian population is so poor that even the reduced premium amounts are too costly and not urgent enough for them to invest. Simultaneously, recent studies have noted that increasingly, even the poorest of families can afford small intermittent contributions, which over a period of time can add up to a significant amount. While the latter may be indicative of emerging trends, the former is a more accurate account of predominant issues facing healthcare financing in India today.

Recognizing this as a major glitch in CBHI schemes, current plans in India have evolved their own *ad hoc* solutions to include the poorest sectors of the populations. For instance, the staff members of Medical Insurance Scheme (MIS) – RAHA pay the premiums for the poorest communities in their field area out of their own pockets. Similarly, ACCORD-AMS-ASHWINI Health Insurance asks for greater premium contributions from those who can afford to help subsidize the premium costs for those who cannot. Finally, in some states and through sparse policies, the government also provides certain subsidies to this section of society. All of these arrangements, however, are improvized, as mentioned, with no formal or sustainable structure in place.

Advancing the Public-Private Partnership

The term Public-Private Partnership (PPP) carries with it a variety of connotations, many of which remain confusing and at times even conflicting. Due to the diverse nature of development schemes in general, PPP programs have taken on multiple forms with various focuses, often redefining its most current explanation. In a general sense, PPP, as it pertains to development, has been defined as "institutional relationships between the state and the private for-profit and/or the private not-for-profit sector, where the different public and private sectors jointly participate in defining the objectives, the methods, and the implementation of an agreement of cooperation" [Jutting: 2000].

However, for the purpose of this study, the not-for-profit sector can be re-characterized as a public actor assuming greater responsibilities in implementing and enforcing social developmental schemes otherwise overseen by the government. Therefore, PPPs can also be defined as institutional relationships between the for-profit private sector and various actors in both the not-for-profit sector and the state-parties that directly work on issues of public concern.

Since the notion of a partnership implies that the parties involved contribute mutually to some ongoing set of interactions aimed to meet a purpose, these same parties must agree to the roles they play within this union. The actors of a PPP can take on one of the three common functions: Provisionary, financial and regulatory and monitory. Those in the provisionary role literally provide a service to the target community, such as healthcare or education. On the other hand, actors assuming the financial role simply help to monetarily support the implementation of the set program. Finally, PPP players who acquire the regulatory and monitory role take responsibility for many administrative tasks required to ensure sustainability and efficiency of the objective [Jutting: 2000].

Leveraging the Public-Private Partnership for Healthcare Financing

Although the discussion regarding PPP in the health sector typically addresses the private and public health delivery mechanisms and ways in which the two can cooperatively provide care, the value of a PPP arrangement can also be utilized to make healthcare financing viable for the rural poor. As enumerated earlier, while CBHI schemes have been the most successful programs in extending the reach of healthcare financing to the poor of India, such plans are still unproductive in insuring the extreme poor populations of the nation. With limited ability to pay for their daily means, individuals and families that fall into this poorest section of society are both unwilling and unable to fund monthly or annual CBHI premiums integral to the mechanism of risk pooling. This inherent malfunction in CBHI schemes can be addressed through the utilization of PPPs.

Riding the momentum of the increasing trend toward corporate social responsibility, corporations all over India have begun to include issues of social concern in their agendas. More and more companies have initiated projects in which administrators allocate resources, both manual and financial, to help advance a social need, such as contributing to funds created for education or health. In some cases, corporations have even established with full committees dedicated to seeking out opportunities for the company to remain actively and continually involved with certain development schemes. Eaton Corporation, in Pune, has established multi-member committees of employees who survey, assess and initiate participation in various developmental projects with NGOs in the area. The same behavior can be leveraged to provide healthcare financing for the rural poor.

Because affordability is a salient issue preventing the rural poor from obtaining CBHI, receiving monetary support from the proximal corporate sector offers an efficient and effective solution. For corporations looking to satisfy their corporate social responsibility, commitment in providing financial support for a project serves as a useful and straightforward mechanism to aid the community. Specifically dealing with healthcare financing, corporations could finance the insurance premia for severely poor families in need of greater access to the health system.

Implementation: The Role of the NGO as an Intermediary

While the above-mentioned PPP appears sound in theory, there are many logistical complications that could make this type of corporate sponsorship program ineffective. NGOs must be appointed as central actors in such a sponsorship program as they are integral to the program's implementation. While the financial means fall within the hands of the corporations, accessibility to the community is a privilege almost exclusively held by the NGO. NGOs are closely linked to rural village communities within which they work. Generally speaking, members of an NGO have worked with the same community for multiple years and have built a rapport and trust that a newcomer would not experience. It is through this fundamental relationship that NGOs are able to help put into practice developmental schemes that rural poor communities would otherwise live without. Combining the strengths of these two major components, the for-profit private sector can come together with the not-for-profit sector through a PPP that can help bring healthcare to the villages.

Working out the various CBHI models, the corporate sponsorship program can take on one of two implementation models: One, where the NGO acts as the intermediary between the insurance provider, the sponsoring corporation, and the communities; and the other, where the NGO actually acts as the insurance provider, and assumes the role as an intermediary between the corporations and the community (see Figure 6).

Literally occupying the central role, NGOs are charged with the responsibility of connecting for-profit funding to the community's health needs, while, in the case of model two, they cooperate with an outside insurance agency. NGOs also may carry administrative duties such as the collection of corporate contributions and the gathering of member information from the rural poor population. The case study presented in the following page outlines the basic features of one such PPP currently being piloted in the Indian state of Maharashtra.

Figure 6: NGOs Serve as the Conduit of PPPs

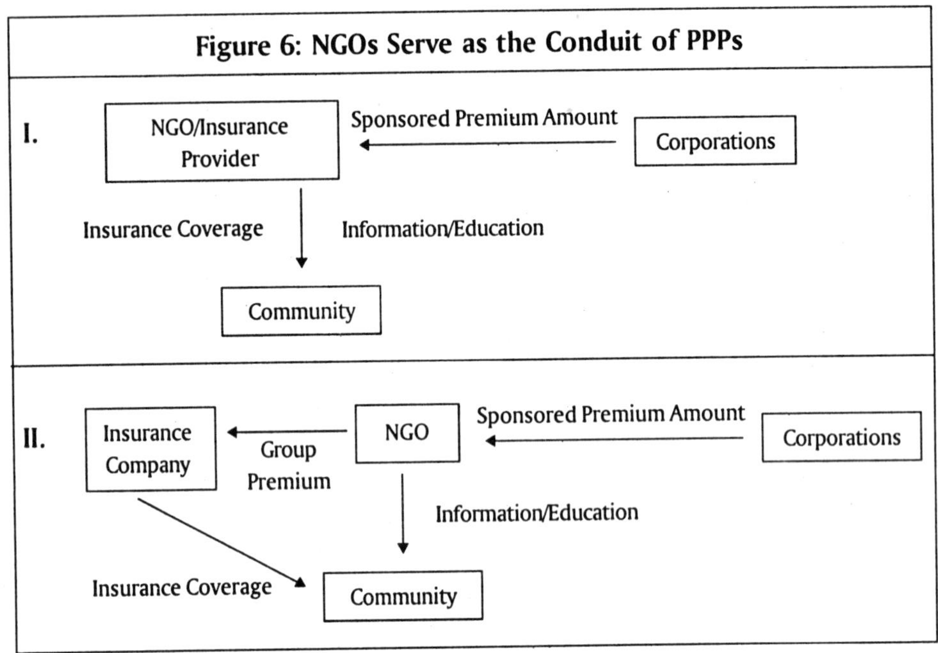

Case Study: Chaitanya and HDFC-Chubb General Insurance

As an example of the above-examined PPP, Chaitanya and HDFC-Chubb General Insurance located in the Pune district of Maharashtra, have recently joined in an endeavor to provide CBHI coverage to SHG-women and their families in the Chaitanya field area. Founded in 1993, Chaitanya focuses on the establishment and strengthening of SHGs and development through microfinance programs. Chaitanya's work has motivated the formation of the Grameen Mahila Swayamsiddha Sangha, the first independent federation of SHGs in Maharashtra. Currently, Chaitanya also carries out developmental activities including water and sanitation, agriculture, livelihood, and health.

HDFC-Chubb General Insurance (GIC)

HDFC Bank and Chubb Corporation, USA entered a venture together in 2002 to jointly offer general insurance services. Specifically, HDFC-Chubb GIC offers a rural initiatives program tailored to meet the needs of the rural poor and offer insurance services at reduced costs.

Rural Initiatives Group Health Insurance Package

- Covers both personal accident and hospitalization expenses.
- Special care and emphasis for women in both personal accident and hospitalization expenses.
- Coverage of husband's accidental death.
- Coverage of permanent disability of the woman member.
- Maternity benefit hospitalization coverage for both normal and cesarean births.
- Compensation of lost wages due to hospitalization.

Table 2: Rural Initiatives Health Insurance Package

Members Insured	Premium (Per family)			
Insured member and spouse only	165	275	385	500
Insured member, spouse, and up to a maximum of two dependent children	220	330	440	600
Insured member, spouse, up to a maximum of two dependent children, and dependent parents	330	495	630	825
Coverage received	7,000	14,000	21,000	28,000

Corporate Sponsorship Program

As a means to help villagers with finance premium costs, Chaitanya and HDFC-Chubb GIC have appealed corporations in the Pune area to become a third link to this PPP, playing a financial role in the partnership. Specifically, representatives have appealed to corporations to encourage corporate employees to participate in a one-to-one sponsorship program where one corporate employee would sponsor the health insurance premium for one specific family in the villages Chaitanya oversees. Money contributed to the scheme first goes to Chaitanya, who then deposits a lump sum into the HDFC-Chubb system. Chaitanya provides the link between HDFC-Chubb, contributing corporations, and the rural villages.

Corporations and NGOs Assess Degree of Involvement

Just as the NGO may play various roles, the corporations involved in this scheme can also participate in more than one manner. For instance, if a corporation believes that this particular funding scheme is one through which it would like to make a long-term commitment, then NGOs can focus on linking up with a few select corporations, who plan to maintain a multiple year partnership with the NGO and its relevant villages. The problem with this plan, however, is that if these few committed corporations fold at some point or back out of the agreement made, the NGO, and the community, would lose a large portion of the premium money, leaving the scheme financially vulnerable. On the other hand, if corporations are not attracted to making long-term funding commitments, NGOs can focus on obtaining a broad base of corporations that regularly contribute. This latter model allows for a continual flow of premium money without incurring significant setbacks, if a corporation were to change its plans. However, it lacks a type of investment in its community that the former model would encourage. Furthermore, following the diversification option, it would require the NGO to consistently and actively create new partnerships while attempting to manage those already existing. Table 3 outlines the advantages and disadvantages of the type of involvement corporations can make.

Table 3: Financial Involvement

Nature of Investment	Duration of Financial Commitment	Consistent Money Flow	Financial Risk	Relationship Maintenance on Part of NGO	Community Investment by Contributor
Few Select Corporations Invest	Long-term	Yes	High	High	High
Many Various Companies Invest	Highly Variable	No	Low	Low	Low

PPP must Include Features to Help Change Mindsets, not Merely Behavior

While the funding of such a scheme is an effective means to initiate CBHI schemes, it is imperative that certain measures are put in place to ensure that villagers' mindsets expand in regard to their understanding and knowledge of healthcare practices. The facilitating of healthcare financing for rural poor should help improve access to the healthcare system, but not without some investment on the part of those receiving its benefit. For this reason, any offering made from the corporate end of the PPP should be partial in its contribution, and with time, taper out (Figure 7). For instance, the first few years that such a PPP manages to successfully enroll and maintain a rural villager membership, the corporate contribution should equal 95% of the premium cost, leaving the remaining 5% onus on the villagers themselves. After the first few years, the corporate contribution should lessen, going from 95% to 80%, then eventually to 50%, etc. incrementally until corporations are providing minimal to no funding for these premia. Ideally speaking, after 5 to 10 years of utilizing a type of healthcare financing scheme, the villagers themselves will find value in the insurance and be willing to finance their own premia. Of course, certain provisions must be made for those families unable to pay for their own premia regardless of their understanding the value of investing in one's health.

Figure 7: Community Investment is Integral to Success of Corporate Sponsorship Scheme

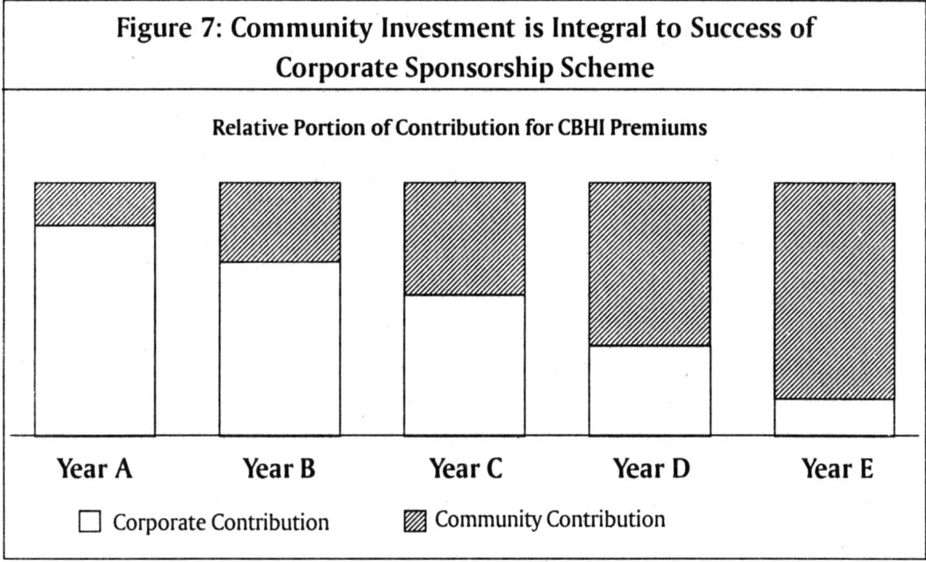

In addition to ensuring that villagers provide some monetary investment in their healthcare, rural poor populations enrolled in the corporate sponsorship PPP must receive regular information regarding the scheme, its purpose, and the importance of sound health habits overall—a task most likely to be delegated to the intermediate NGO. Healthcare financing must serve not only as a means for the poor to gain access to the health system, but also as a tool through which rural populations gain a greater understanding about preventive health practices and why habitual investments in one's health today will save more money in the future. Corporate financing of this scheme is a means through which healthcare financing can be made possible for the poor, but it should not be a permanent fixture in their lives.

Conclusion

Developmental schemes to curb the poverty cycle are numerous and each is distinct in its approach to mobilizing unprivileged communities. Development in the health sector is one of the most basic areas through which rural poor populations of developing nations, such as India, can gain ground in advancing their community. The lack of adequate healthcare for these groups originates from their lack of education as well as from poor healthcare infrastructure in the nation. The disproportionate amount of private health spending to that of public spending in India places the burden of healthcare in the hands of the every individual, expenditure that are often too expensive for average households to shoulder, let alone for the poorer segments of society. As this article details, the most viable and present solution to improve people's healthcare access in India, while making financing affordable, is to invest in CBHI schemes tailored to provide basic healthcare to those without cover. As a means to ensure effective and efficient implementation of CBHI schemes, the private and public sectors should come together in a joint project through which the rural poor can receive health coverage through the reallocation of capital.

(Sudha Menon is Consulting Editor at the Icfai Research Centre, Ahmedabad. She can be reached at sudhamenon@yahoo.co.in).

13

Community-Based Hospital
An Alternative Healthcare Arrangement for the Rural Poor in West Bengal

Srabanti Chakravarti and Kaushik Chakraborty

This article focuses on the perception of the rural masses of West Bengal about health and the ways of medical treatment. The authors have clearly segregated the entire database into four distinct clusters where the findings depict that cluster four—the most vulnerable group of population—urgently requires a community-based hospital to take care of their health needs. Therefore, it identifies the need of the 5As framework to ensure that the most vulnerable section of the society can participate and benefit from a community-based hospital. In fact, this article is just an isolated attempt for planning five hypothetical model hospitals for which the community members need to contribute Rs.15 per month. If this model is successful, it can be extended to all the districts in West Bengal.

Source: The Icfai Journal of Public Administration, April 2006.

World Health Organization defined health as, "a state of complete physical, mental and social well-being and not merely the absence of disease or infirmity" (1994). On the other hand, health can be defined negatively, as the absence of illness; functionally, as the ability to cope with everyday activities, or positively, as fitness and well-being. In any organism, health is a form of homeostasis. This is a state of balance, with inputs and outputs of energy and matter in equilibrium (allowing for growth). Health also implies good prospects for continued survival. In sentient creatures such as humans, health is a broader concept.[1] "Healthcare" means preventive, diagnostic, therapeutic, rehabilitative, maintenance or palliative care, services, procedures or counselling, including appropriate assistance with disease or symptom management and maintenance, that affects an individual's physical, mental or behavioral condition, including individual cells or their components or genetic information, or affects the structure or function of the human body or any part of the human body...(WHO, 1994.) It may be safely stated that, the wealth of a country is judged by the health of its people. Worldwide, nations are seeking viable answers to the question of how to offer a healthcare system, which leads to improvement in the health status of their citizens. In our opinion, the healthcare in the rural West Bengal is the responsibility of the community as a whole. A collaborative approach, which involves financial support, strategic planning, and health prioritizing legislation involves the government, community leaders, and private and public healthcare professionals. The faults of the medical system of West Bengal have become apparent in the last decade as financial constraints forced hospitals to run with inadequate infrastructure facilities in the hospital care system and reducing staff, thereby reducing patients' access to timely services. Moreover, ambulatory services or, in other words, the patients' transportation services in rural West Bengal are in a precarious condition. From years of evidence, public and private healthcare understands the need to view healthcare from a nation's development perspective; however, without losing sight of the need to provide high quality and accessible services. Indeed, one must strive to improve the healthcare system by creating an environment that encourages and rewards quality of care by the professionals providing the services. As a standard, all the people of rural West Bengal should have access to healthcare and supportive services. Through tightly coordinated partnerships with medical, social, civic and religious organizations of this country,

1 *en.wikipedia.org/wiki/Health*

one can develop a comprehensive and coordinated healthcare system, a system, which relies on community leadership and community inputs and focuses on preventing diseases rather than treating avoidable complications. By tapping into interdisciplinary services, one can concentrate on the prevention of common public health problems, such as diarrhea, Kala Azar, Malaria, Arsenic problems, jaundice and other problems, thereby reducing the incidence and complications of disease and illness. Besides, the surgery cases also require specialist services. Perhaps, this is the forum to highlight the priority of health for our citizens, within the realm of development of the government's infrastructure and guidance from the various ministries involved in education, health and community development. Quality healthcare must be a right of all the people of the rural West Bengal.

In this article, the authors make an attempt to analyze the perception of the rural people of West Bengal about the quality of healthcare provided to them. The objective of this paper is also to find out why the existing system of health centers as a vehicle of healthcare service provider has almost failed to make significant impact on the rural masses of West Bengal and to develop a viable model of making the healthcare available and accessible to the rural masses of West Bengal.

Methodology

The proposed study is based on both primary and secondary data. Secondary data has been collected from different journals and related web sites (mentioned in the references and many more), information available with the insurance companies, statistics collected by the government, trade associations and other non-governmental development agencies. Primary data is collected from some selected villages of West Bengal. A structured questionnaire is administered to respondents in the course of survey. In this study, the researchers employed Cluster analysis by using SPSS* to identify the homogeneous consumer segments among the Indian rural masses for utilizing the healthcare services and its financing mechanisms available in India. This procedure assumes that the data falls into a known number of clusters. Given this number, the procedure will assign cases to clusters. One can select one of the two methods to classify cases, i.e., either update cluster centers iteratively or classify only. The outcome of the process is cluster memberships, distance information and final cluster centers.

---

* Statistical Package for Social Sciences.

Exhibit 1: Sampling Unit – Some Selected Villages of West Bengal

District	Villages
Bankura	Brahmandiha, Gaurbazar, Indpur, Hatogram, Brajorajpur, Raghunathpur, Khatra Gram 1
Hooghly	Siakhala, Mashat, Patul, Harirambati, Jangipara
South 24-Paraganas	Dakshin Barashat, Usti, Nurpur, Dhamua

Sample size: Since this is just a pilot survey, the authors surveyed 100 households as per convenience sampling method.

Facts and Findings

The k means cluster analysis by using SPSS 10.0 has clearly classified the entire database into four meaningful clusters. The features of each cluster are as follows:

Cluster 1

Cluster 1 comprises 6% of the total respondents. The cluster is literate and the average qualification of the cluster is beyond the secondary level. The respondents by occupation are school teachers, rural doctors, government service holders, businessmen, land owners etc. The average age of the cluster is 49 and average household income is Rs.10,167. The average number of dependents is two. The cluster strongly denied that they have a sound health. They admitted that they know the leading causes of diseases in their locality, but they could not respond to the aspect of preventive measures to avoid bracing the diseases. The *Anganwadi* workers normally do not visit them or even try to motivate them. When they are sick, they normally go to the nearest town for checkup. They did not agree to visit the rural health centers even when they are sick. However, they agreed to visit rural private practitioners during urgency. They normally believe in allopathic treatment. They never visit the quacks for treatment. The respondents opined that the village health centers are not well equipped. According to them, the doctors of the health centers are well trained but due to lack of infrastructure, they are unable to provide proper service. They strongly disagreed that any surgical operations can be conducted with the medical infrastructure available in the rural areas. They stated that they do not have any arrangements to transport patients to the nearest towns. However, they refer the patients to private ambulatory services. The respondents also claimed that though these ambulatory services are limited and costly, it is affordable to them. In the villages the respondents do not have pathological setups for blood test and urine culture, etc. They said that the villages are devoid of X-ray clinics or sonography facilities. They comfortably bear their medical expenses. They disagreed that they need to take loans for their catastrophic medical expenses. They strongly disagreed on the point that they need to sell assets for their unforeseen medical expenses. They stated that they never availed a charitable monetary help from their relatives or acquaintances in case of catastrophic medical expenses. They are in favor of private nursing homes for their treatment. They don't want community-based hospitals run by their own community for their treatment. From the questionnaire, it is evident that they do not agree to contribute Rs.15 per month for the development of community-based hospital. However, apart from the questionnaire, from the discussion the researchers had, it was evident that some of them agreed to provide some philanthropic grant for building up such hospital for the poor.

Cluster 2

Cluster 2 comprises 12% of the total respondents. The cluster is literate and the average qualification of the cluster is just below the secondary education level. The respondents, by occupation, are primary schoolteachers, Group D staff of the Government, casual labor, small businessmen, farmers working in their own land, etc. The average age of the cluster is 40 and average household income is Rs.4,042. The average number of dependents is three. The cluster denied that they have a sound health. The cluster kept undecided on the issue that they know the leading causes of diseases in their locality. They denied taking any preventive measures to protect themselves from the leading causes of diseases. The *Anganwadi* workers normally do not visit them to make them aware of the health hazards. Their health conditions are not that good and most of them need treatment within a year. They were undecided on transporting the patients to the nearby towns. They denied going to the rural health centers for checkup. They were undecided on going to the rural private practitioners for checkup. They said that if they were sick, they would not depend on alternative medical treatment, like homeopathy, which costs much less than allopathic treatment. They denied going to the rural quacks for treatment. They said that the villages do not have ray clinics or sonography facilities. They denied that they bear the medical expenses comfortably. They kept undecided on the question of taking loan for unforeseen medical expenses. How then do they meet the expenses? They were also confused on whether they need charitable monetary help from their relatives or acquaintances in case of catastrophic medical expenses and in question of charitable organizations to take initiative for medical care. They raise loans to meet the medical expenses. They do not want community-based hospitals managed by Ramakrishna Mission, Bharat *Sevashram Sangha,* etc. Therefore, they do not agree to contribute Rs.15 per month for development of a community-based hospital.

Cluster 3

Cluster 3 comprises of 3% of the total respondents. The cluster is literate and the average qualification of the cluster is above the secondary education level. The respondents by occupation are rich businessmen, big landowners, retired government employees, etc. The average age of the cluster is 50 and average household income is Rs.17,333 per month. The average number of dependents is one. They state that they do not have good health since one or the other problem is always there. They know the leading causes of diseases in their locality. However, they do not take any preventive measures against those diseases. They denied that the *Anganwadi* workers do not visit them and make them aware of the preventive measures against the leading causes of diseases. They strongly denied that their health condition is good and therefore require medical checkups frequently in a year. They state that they go to the nearest town for medical checkup. They denied visiting rural health centers at the time of illness. They visit the rural private practitioners at the time of illness. When sick, they would not depend on alternative medical treatment, like homeopathy, which costs much less than the allopathic treatment. They never go to the quacks at the time of illness. They agreed that the rural health centers are not at all well equipped. According to them, the doctors of the health centers are well trained but due to lack of infrastructure, they are unable to provide proper medical services. They agreed that any surgical operations could be conducted by the medical infrastructure of rural areas. They said that the ambulatory services for patient transportation is a must. The patient transportation facilities are limited but not beyond their means. In the villages, the respondents do not have pathological lab for blood test, urine culture etc. They said that the villages are devoid of X-ray clinics or sonography facilities. They comfortably bear their medical expenses. They need not go for loans, sell assets or take charitable monetary help from their relatives. They are in favor of private nursing homes in their locality for their treatment. They are of the opinion that any charitable organization run community hospital would serve their purpose. From the questionnaire, it is evident that they do not agree to contribute Rs.15 per month for development of the community-based hospital. However, apart from the questionnaire, from the discussion the researchers had with them, it was evident that some of them agree to provide some philanthropic grant for building up such a hospital for the poor.

Cluster 4

Cluster 4 is the biggest cluster comprising 79% of the total respondents. Most of the respondents of this cluster are illiterate. Their maximum education level is class VI. The respondents, by occupation, are marginal farmers, farmers cultivating on their own land and artisans etc. The average age of the cluster is 39 and average household income is Rs.970. The average number of dependents is three. The respondents denied that they have good health. They do not know the leading causes of diseases in their locality. They do not take any preventive measures against the leading causes of diseases in their locality. They have no faith on the rural health centers to get cured of their illness. They are unable to pay the private practitioners and hence they do not consult them at the time of illness. They depend on homeopathic, ayurvedic or other low-cost treatment. They stated that they visit the rural quarks at the time of illness. They denied that the rural health centers are well equipped. They also claimed that the doctors of the health centers are well trained but due to lack of infrastructure, they are unable to provide proper medical services. They said that it is not possible to conduct surgical cases in their locality. They denied having access to any ambulatory facility. They agreed that although there are limited ambulatory services in their locality, they are beyond their reach. In the villages, the respondents do not have pathological setups for blood test, urine culture etc. They said that the villages do not have X-ray clinics or sonography facilities. They denied bearing catastrophic medical expenses comfortably. They agreed to take loans to bear catastrophic medical expenses. However, they refused to talk about the question of selling assets to bear the catastrophic medical expenses. They agreed that they take charitable monetary help from their relatives. They do not want any private nursing homes for their treatment. They want community-based hospitals run by their own community. They have no problem if such a hospital is managed by Ramakrishna Mission, Bharat *Sevashram Sangha,* etc. They agreed to contribute Rs.15 per month for development of community-based hospital, as it was a good solution to their burning problem.

The Proposed Solution – Community-Based Hospital

The above discussion clearly suggests that the clusters 1,2,3 are not agreeable to the proposal of community-based hospital. However, cluster 4, which is the most vulnerable group of population, urgently requires a community-based hospital to take care of their health hazards. Therefore, the story considers the 5As framework that needs to be addressed to ensure that most vulnerable section of the society can participate in and benefit from community-based hospital. The concept of 5As refers to:

- **Availability:** Rural health centres are at least 3 km away from the surveyed areas. Nursing homes are hardly found. In some of the villages, private clinical laboratories are just opened. Medical stores are found in developed villages. Some important emergency drugs, saline bottles and oxygen cylinders are not found in these stores. There are no blood banks in the rural areas. The health centres ensure the establishment and implementation of a comprehensive Human Resource Strategy, which includes the development and training of staff in health promotion skills. In sub centres only one ANM* staff nurse reports. On many occasions, the health centres do not have adequate number of doctors. Doctors, staying in the cities, that are posted to the rural health centers, visit once or twice a week. Moreover, there are no specialist doctors in the sub centers. In this situation, the poor villagers have to depend on local quacks, which results in dangers. The equipment available is just the delivery kits etc. Besides this, the health

* Auxiliary Nurse Midwife.

centers fail to provide basic amenities and drugs to the patients due to scanty supplies. In the health centres, there is no provision for basic clinical tests like X-ray, blood test, ultrasonography, etc. There is no proper infrastructure for surgical cases. In this situation, to ensure the availability of healthcare services to the BPL[+] population, there is a need for full-fledged low-cost rural hospitals from where they can avail of these services.

- **Accessibility:** It is very difficult for the poorest to transport the patient in absence of ambulance. The only means for patient transportation is the rickshaw van by which it is difficult to transport serious patients in poor road conditions, especially during the rainy season. They do not have access to the hospitals in the cities because of the transportation problem and the money involved in transportation of patients, including the fear of negligence. It is better to have five (5) community-based hospitals in a single district. Each hospital can meet the medical needs of all the BPL population within 10-kilometer radius. Moreover, the community-based hospitals should have proper ambulatory services to transport the emergency cases to the hospitals.

- **Affordability:** The nature of rural poverty is quite different from the urban poverty. Rural poor are mainly the landless farmers and craftsman. In some cases, the per capita income is less than Rs.500. In most of the cases, they do not have money for buying allopathic medicines and blood transfusion apart from oxygen cylinder because of acute poverty. The infrastructure of rural hospitals is inadequate for conducting surgical cases and the small nursing homes in the semi-urban areas are totally out of reach to them because of the high costs of treatment. Similar is the case with the newborn clinical laboratories in the rural areas.

- **Awareness:** The rural poor in most of the cases have resigned to their fate. In some cases, they believe in superstitions and seek relief from nonmedical means such as 'jalpara', 'telpara'** etc. Many children did not get polio vaccine because their parents are suspicious about the effect of the vaccine. This psychological inertia is possibly due to illiteracy, ignorance and neglect

+ Below Poverty line.

** A sort of black magic.

of the society that the poor people are subjected to from time immemorial. Therefore the immediate need is to ensure that ten community friends will work under an officer of the hospital to create awareness among the rural masses to become a member of community-based hospitals.

- **Appropriateness:** The above analysis and observations focus on the need of intervention of community-based hospital in the arena of universal access of healthcare and healthcare financing. Although 75% of India's population lives in rural areas, there are considerable inequalities in terms of educational achievements, employment opportunities, purchasing power, and health and its attributes including infant mortality, general morbidity, economic security in terms of assured income earning opportunities and so on. In a small pilot survey carried out in the selected villages of West Bengal, the researchers found that most of the rural peasantry and artisans suffer from malnutrition and chronic diseases associated with acute poverty and poor living conditions. These illnesses keep them off from employment, leading them further into debt trap. As the quantum of access to healthcare in West Bengal villages is quite low and there is a positive correlation between the health improvement and poverty reduction, there is always the need for alternative arrangements. One possible way to combat this situation could be to build up a hypothetical hospital model where universal coverage could be achieved. The researchers suggest a proposal to develop an organization, which will be managed by a trust (formed under Sections *11-13A of Indian Income Tax Act, 1961*) and exempts from paying tax. The authors attempted to develop this model for a single model district South 24 Paraganas where the rural population below poverty line is 3,88,033 families (source: *www.kolkata.wb.nic.in*: downloaded on 9/8/05). In fact, researchers suggest a model hospital for which community members need to contribute Rs.15 per month. After the initial cost of establishment is covered, one can plan for increasing the number of such community-based hospitals. If this model is successful, it can be extended to all the districts in West Bengal in future. The basic assumptions behind the model are, among the total 3,88,033 rural BPL families in south 24 Paraganas, at least 3,00,000 would be motivated by the community friends to become members of the hospitals.

Table 1: Financial Model of 500-Bed Hospital for the below Poverty Line People of Rural South 24 Paraganas

(The Total BPL Population is 3,88,033)

* All the benefits are restricted to the members (contributing Rs.15 per month per family only)

Initial Cash Inflow in the First Year:

Sl. No.	Items	Amount (in Rs.)
1.	Contribution of 3,00,000 @ Rs.15 per month	5,40,00,000
2.	Philanthropic grants	5,00,000
3.	Government grants	10,00,000
	Total Income Per Year	5,55,00,000

Non Recurring Expenditure

1.	**Building Construction**		10,00,000
2.	**Two Operation Theaters**		
	1.	OT tables (2) @ 50,000	1,00,000
	2.	OT lights (2 sets) @ 50,000	1,00,000
	3.	Sucker machines (2) @ 30,000	60,000
	4.	Pulse oxymeters (2) @ 50,000	1,00,000
	5.	Cardiac monitors (2) @ 35,000	70,000
	6.	Boyle's machines with full set (2) @ 1,50,000	3,00,000
	7.	Diathermy machines (2) @ 50,000	1,00,000
	8.	View box (2) @ 1000	2,000
	9.	Autoclave machine (1) @ 1,00,000	1,00,000
	10.	Laryngoscope & endotracheal tube with forceps (2 sets) @ 10,000	20,000
	11.	Other equipment including trolleys	2,00,000
	12.	Furniture, linen and dressings	25,000
3.	**Three Wards (Male 50 Beds, Female 45 Beds, 5 Emergency Beds)**		
	1.	Beds @1500	1,50,000
	2.	Sucker machines (3) @ 30,000	1,20,000
	3.	Pulse oxymeters (3) @ 50,000	1,50,000
	4.	Cardiac monitors (3) @ 35,000	1,05,000
	5.	Nebulisers (2) @ 2,500	5,000
	6.	Others (rail chords, baby chords, kidney trays, trolleys, etc.)	60,000

Contd...

Contd...		
4.	**Labor Room**	
	1. Labor table	5,000
	2. Weighing Machine	1,000
	3. Blood pressure instrument	1,000
	4. Delivery kit	5,000
	5. Other equipment including trolleys	5,000
5.	**OPD Setup**	
	1. Basic equipment	1,00,000
	2. Dental setup	2,00,000
	3. Gynae setup	2,000
6.	**Miscellenous**	
	1. Pathology laboratory	2,00,000
	2. Ambulance	2,50,000
	3. Generator	25,000
	4. Waste disposal containers as directed by Pollution Board	5,000
	Total Non Recurring Expenditure	**35,66,000**

Initial Cash Outflow for Each Hospital

Sl. No.	Items	Amount (in Rs.)
1.	**Recurring Expenditure**	
	Salary of Physician (MBBS) @ 10,000	1,20,000
	Salary of Surgeon (MD) (Doctor-in-charge) @ 15,000	1,80,000
	Salary of anesthetist @ 8,000	96,000
	Salary of gynecologist @ 10,000	1,20,000
	Salary of three part-time specialists (dentist, ENT, osteopath) visiting once a week @ 1,000	36,000
	Salary of pathologist @ 10,000	1,20,000
2.	Salaries of five nurses @ 6,000	3,60,000
	Salary of sister-in charge @ 7,000	84,000
	Salary of store keeper @ 2,500	30,000
3.	Salary of ambulance driver @ 2,000	24,000
	Salaries of peons, ayahs (4) @ 1,000	48,000
		Contd...

Contd...		
	Salary of linen keeper @ 1,000	12,000
	Salary of two sweepers @ 300	7,200
4.	Salary of the Accounts Officer @ 15,000	1,80,000
	Salary of officer (collection) @ 5,000	60,000
	Salary of officer (Investment) @ 5,000	60,000
	Salary of ten community friends @ 2,000	2,40,000
5.	Medicines, saline bottles with saline stands, oxygen cylinders with stands, dressing sets	3,50,000
6.	Transporting patients	2,00,000
7.	Miscellaneous expenses (electric bills, stationery, etc.)	50,000
8.	Depreciation cost (assumed @ 10%)	3,56,600
	Total Recurring Expenditure for Each Hospital	**27,33,800**

Total Expenditure = {Total Non Recurring expenditure + Total Recurring Expenditure + Contingency fund (Rs.5,00,000)} * 5 [as the model is of building five such hospitals]

= {Rs.(35,66,000 + 27,33,800 + 5,00,000)} * 5 = Rs.(67,99,800*5)

= Rs.3,39,99,000

Initial cost for fund generation is assumed to be Rs.10,00,000

Balance = Rs.(5,55,00,000-3,49,99,000)

= Rs.2,05,01,000

This balance amount will be invested for the sustainability of the project.

The Payback Period

The Payback period measures the time required to recover the initial outflow of the project. It is the simplest way of looking at one or more major project ideas. It tells how long it will take to earn back the money spent on the project.

The payback methods is suggested because:

- The project has a deep social impact and deals with human lives. Therefore, its costs and benefits cannot be quantified in monetary terms.

Therefore, in this case, it may be of interest to find out how quickly one can recover the initial investment made.

- The quality of decision-making would be relatively easier in this case than to evaluate under Net Present Value method, internal rate of return method or the other investment evaluative criteria.

Payback period of the project = Initial Outflow/Constant Annual Inflow

= 2,03,30,000/4,03,31,000 years

= 0. 0.50 years (rounded)

= 0.50 * 12 months

= 6 months

Where,

- Initial outflow = Total Non Recurring expenditure + Contingency Fund + Initial cost for fund generation.
- Constant Annual Inflow = Annual Contribution by Members – Yearly Recurring Expenditure.

Generally, a payback period of three years or less is preferred. Some advisors opine that if the payback period is less than a year, the project should be considered essentials. (*see www.toolkit.cch.com*). Therefore, as per the Payback period method, initial investment of the concerning project could be recovered within six months, i.e., less than even a year. Therefore, the project is not only viable but also quite essential.

Investment Portfolio

In this project, Rs.2,05,01,000 remains as surplus at the end of the first year, which can be invested in several investment schemes. If one assumes a flat 8% rate of interest per annum, then, by next year, an additional Rs.16,40,080 would be generated, which can cover the major portion of annual recurring expenditure. In that case, the subscription rate of members can be reduced further in future.

Conclusion

Although 75% of India's population lives in rural areas, there are notable inequalities in terms of their educational achievements, employment opportunities, purchasing power, health and its attributes including infant mortality, general morbidity, economic security in terms of assured income earning opportunities and so on. In a phase-wise survey carried out in the selected villages of West Bengal, it is found that most of the rural peasantry and artisans suffer from malnutrition and chronic diseases associated with acute poverty and poor living conditions. These illnesses keep them off employment, leaving them to further debt. As the quantum of access to healthcare in the villages of West Bengal is quite low and there is a positive correlation between the health improvement and poverty reduction, there is always the need for alternative healthcare arrangements. One possible way to combat this situation could be making healthcare coverage available and accessible to the below poverty line population keeping community-based hospital as the nodal agency. However, this is just a simple attempt, which definitely cannot be conclusive. Moreover, the database is very small and so the chance of oversimplification or bias cannot be ruled out. Nevertheless, this attempt would definitely be a torchbearer to the researchers involved in this area of study.

(Srabanti Chakravarti, Assistant Professor, IIAS School of Management, Kolkata,

Kaushik Chakraborty, Research Associate, The Icfai National College, Regional Office, Kolkata.)

Annexure: Questionnaire

Name: Age: Sex:

Occupation: Income: No. of dependent family members:

Education: Average healthcare expense per month:

1. Strongly Agree 2. Agree 3. Can't decide 4. Disagree 5. Strongly Disagree

Sl	Questions (Attributes)	1	2	3	4	5
1	You understand the concept of good health (5)					
2	You know the leading causes of diseases in your locality (6)					
3	You know the causes of diseases in your locality and take precautionary measures to handle those (7)					
4	Your local *Anganwadi* workers or health center employees made you aware of the health-related matters (8)					
5	Your health condition is good and you didn't need any check-up since last one year (9)					
6	If you are sick, you will go to the nearest town for treatment (10)					
7	If you are sick, you will go to the rural health center for treatment (11)					
8	If you are sick, you will go to rural private practitioner for treatment (12)					
9	If you are sick, you will depend on alternative medical treatment like homeopathy, which costs much less than allopathic treatment (13)					
10	If you are sick, you will go to quacks for treatment (14)					
11	Your village health center is not well equipped (15)					
12	The rural health centers are equipped, but they are devoid of health practitioners (16)					
13	It is possible to conduct surgical cases in your village (17)					
14	You don't have any arrangement to transport patients to the nearest town hospital in your locality (18)					
15	You have limited arrangements to transport patients and those are very costly and beyond your capacity (19)					
16	In your village, you have pathological setup for blood test, urine culture etc. (20)					
17	You have X-ray clinic and ultrasonography facilities at reasonable rates in your village (21)					
18	You can bear your medical expenses comfortably (22)					
19	You need to take loan for your catastrophic medical expenses (23)					
20	You need to sell assets for your catastrophic medical expenses (24)					

Contd...

Contd...		
21	You will need charitable monetary help from your relatives or acquaintances in case of catastrophic medical expenses (25)	
22	You want private nursing homes for your treatment (26)	
23	You want community-based hospitals run by your own community (27)	
24	You want community-based hospital managed by Ramakrishna Mission, Bharat *Sevashram Sangha* etc. (28)	
25	You want to contribute Rs.15 per family for developing a community hospital where you will get all free ambulatory and hospital services (both in patient and out patient) (29)	

Initial Cluster Centers

	Cluster			
	1	2	3	4
V1	55	45	58	35
V2	10000	5000	20000	150
V3	2	1	1	1
V5	5	5	5	4
V6	3	3	3	4
V7	4	5	5	5
V8	5	5	5	5
V9	4	5	5	5
V10	1	5	1	5
V11	4	5	5	5
V12	3	3	3	4
V13	5	5	5	4
V14	5	5	5	4
V15	3	5	1	5
V16	5	5	5	5
V17	5	5	5	5
V18	5	5	5	1
V19	5	5	5	1
V20	1	5	4	5
V21	1	5	4	5
V22	1	5	1	5
V23	5	5	5	1
V24	5	5	5	4
V25	5	5	5	1
V26	1	5	1	5
V27	5	5	5	1
V28	5	5	5	5
V29	5	4	4	1

Final Cluster Centers

	Cluster			
	1	2	3	4
V1	49	40	50	39
V2	10167	4042	17333	970
V3	2	3	1	3
V5	5	4	5	3
V6	2	3	2	4
V7	3	4	5	4
V8	5	4	5	2
V9	4	4	5	4
V10	2	3	1	4
V11	4	4	5	4
V12	2	3	2	4
V13	4	4	5	2
V14	5	4	5	2
V15	1	2	1	3
V16	5	4	5	2
V17	5	5	5	4
V18	4	3	4	2
V19	4	3	4	2
V20	4	3	1	4
V21	4	3	1	4
V22	2	4	1	5
V23	4	3	4	2
V24	5	4	5	3
V25	4	3	4	2
V26	2	3	1	4
V27	4	3	4	2
V28	5	4	5	2
V29	4	4	4	2

Number of Cases in Each Cluster

Cluster	1	6.000
	2	12.000
	3	3.000
	4	79.000
Valid		100.000
Missing		.000

14

The Farmer Field School
A Method for Enhancing the Role of Rural Communities in Malaria Control?

Henk van den Berg and Bart GJ Knols

Malaria has strong linkages with agriculture, and farmers in malarious regions have a central position in creating or controlling the conditions that favour disease transmission. An interdisciplinary and integrated approach is needed to involve farmers and more than one sector in control efforts. It is suggested that malaria control can benefit from a complementary intervention in rural development—the Farmer Field School (FFS) on Integrated Pest Management (IPM). This is a form of education that uses experiential learning methods to build farmers' expertise, and has proven farm-level and empowerment effects. The benefits of incorporating malaria control into the IPM curriculum are discussed. An example of a combined health-agriculture curriculum, labeled Integrated Pest and Vector Management (IPVM), developed in Sri Lanka is presented. Institutional ownership and support for IPVM could potentially be spread over several public sectors requiring a process for institutional learning and reform.

Source: Malaria Journal 2006, 5:3 (www.malariajournal.com).

Introduction

Malaria has major and multifaceted linkages with agriculture, both in a rural and peri-urban context [1,2]. Agricultural environments provide conditions well suited for anopheline breeding, with clear, temporary water bodies coinciding with the time of crop cultivation, and human and animal hosts at flying distance. Clearing of land for agriculture opens up breeding habitats for heliophilic vectors, whereas "informal" smallholder farming systems located near natural water sources, such as streams and rivers, open up vector breeding opportunities. Moreover, mounting evidence indicates that the widespread agricultural use of broad-spectrum insecticides contributes to insecticide-resistance in mosquito vectors [3,4]. This is expected to reduce the efficacy of indoor residual spraying and insecticide-treated bednets, although the efficacy of the latter intervention has, so far, only been marginally unaffected even in areas with high frequency of the *kdr* gene in the vector population [5]. In addition, agriculture generates income and, thus, influences living conditions, which can affect the transmission and severity of disease. Malaria, in turn, impedes human workforce output and agricultural production, especially at times that agricultural activities peak (i.e., the time of irrigation or after rains). In the African context, this effect is exemplified by the dual role of women in agricultural activities and as family caregiver.

Central in all these crucial linkages is the position of farmers – who create the agricultural environments, implement the cultivation practices, decide on agrochemical inputs, and who attain, as a result of these actions, a certain living standard. Addressing the malaria-agriculture interface requires, therefore, a broad interdisciplinary and integrated approach that involves local communities and more than one public sector. The importançe of active participation and empowerment of rural communities to the effectiveness of malaria control interventions and to the sustainability of their outcomes has been repeatedly stressed [6]. Some progress has been made by making health services better embedded within community structures [7,8] or marketing systems [9], but these developments do not necessarily result in local initiative or the empowerment of communities.

In the area of environmental management, which is receiving renewed interest, past project attempts have shown that it can be difficult to motivate local people into action [10], possibly, as has been suggested, due to the absence of economic incentive

Figure 1

The FFS activity of Agro-Ecosystem Analysis Depicted, with the Stages of (a) Regular Field Observation, (b) Drawing and Analysis, and (c) Presentation and Group Discussion

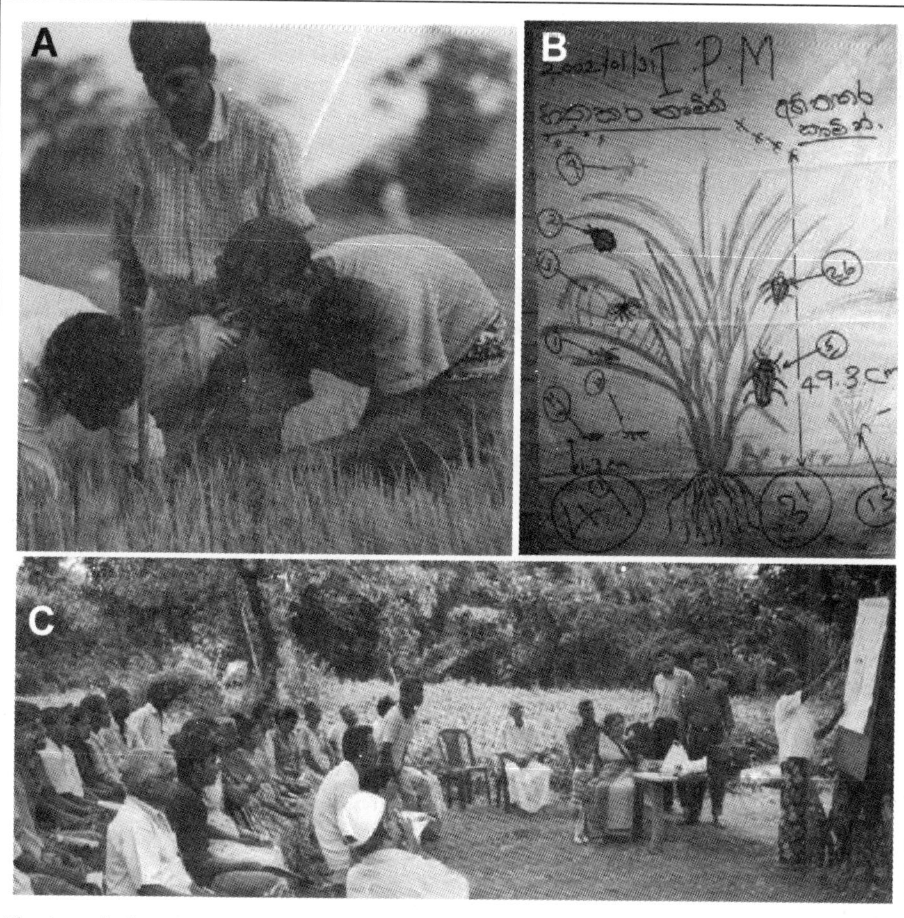

Photographs by H Van Den Berg, Sri Lanka, 2002.

mechanisms [6]. There have been examples of successful initiatives [11-13], but their sustainability remains an issue. Evidently, experience with participation and empowerment of rural people is most established within the agricultural sector. A variety of interpretations of participation exist, ranging from passive participation (where people are told what is to happen) and functional participation (as a means to achieve external goals), to self-mobilization (where the people take initiative), with the latter most likely to lead to positive change [14]. In this commentary, the potential value of a popular participatory approach for malaria control, called the Farmer Field School, is discussed, while drawing on experience from a project in Sri Lanka.

Figure 2

Four possible effects of IPVM Farmer Field Schools on malaria disease: (a) the effect of reduced agro-pesticide use on the risk of insecticide resistance in vector mosquitoes; (b) the effect of increased awareness and understanding about malaria on personal protection measures and treatment-seeking behaviour; (c) the effect of increased profits from agriculture on nutrition and housing conditions; (d) the effect of environmental management on vector breeding and thus on the transmission of disease.

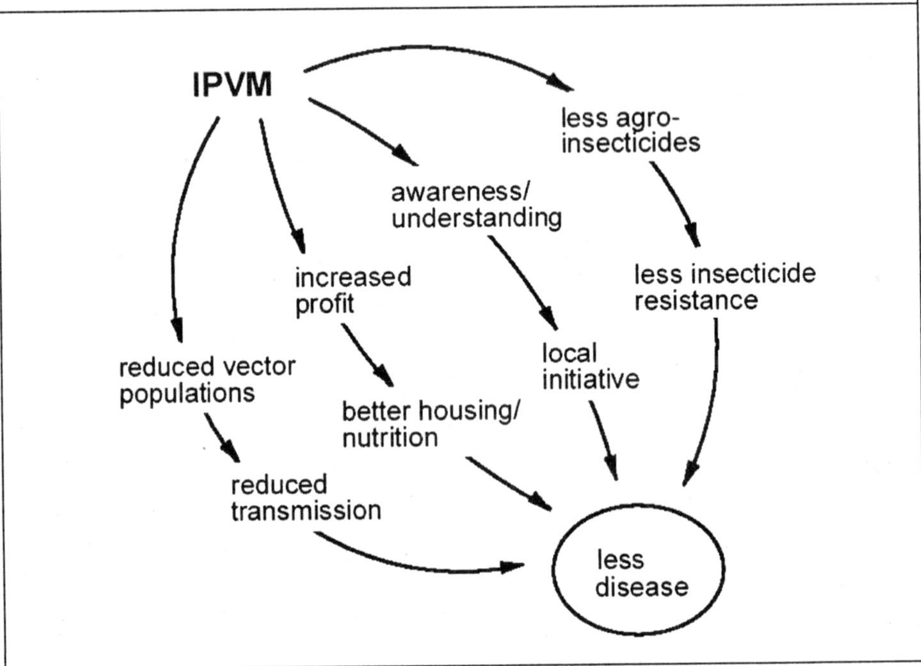

Farmer Field School

The Farmer Field School (FFS) has one of the most impressive track records in participatory community approaches [15], with 2-3 million farmers graduated on the agricultural subject of Integrated Pest Management (IPM) during the past 15 years, mainly in Asia, but more recently also in Africa, the Middle East and Latin America [16]. A review of 25 impact studies indicated a range of positive outcomes of IPM Farmer Field Schools including drastic reductions in agro-pesticide use, economic benefits and empowerment effects [17]. The FFS approach evolved from the need to strengthen the ecological basis of Integrated Pest Management (IPM) to deal with the variability and complexity of agro-ecosystems whilst reducing reliance on pesticides. The ecology of opportunist insects (which include mosquitoes) is highly localized and dynamic, with populations fluctuating manyfold both spatially and temporally. Accordingly, most tropical smallholder agro-ecosystems require management decisions that are tailored to local and contemporary conditions. This implies the need to decentralize expertise to the field level by educating local people to analyse field situations and to make appropriate management decisions.

The Farmer Field School is a form of education which uses experiential learning methods to build farmers' expertise [18]. In sessions at weekly intervals during a crop cycle, a group of 15-30 neighbouring farmers meet in an open-air situation to take observations of the agro-ecosystem (Figure 1). Several sub-groups of farmers sample the populations and characteristics of harmful and beneficial organisms, plants, soil and environmental conditions. These observations are analysed and presented on newsprint for group discussion, which provides an opportunity for speculation (for example, "what if, instead of spraying, we drain the water to control planthoppers in rice"), leading to decision-making on experimental action to be evaluated in the following week. These weekly completed learning cycles result in strengthened skills and increased confidence of farmers. Several additional observations or experiments are conducted during the field school to study life cycles, insect behaviour, and plant damage. Group dynamics and communication exercises are conducted to strengthen group cohesion, maintain motivation and help participants to develop organizational skills. Group building is important in approaches such as IPM and disease vector management, which benefit from coordinated management by many farmers over a large area. Post FFS support has been given in a number of countries to facilitate the emergence of local project initiative [18].

Multi-Pronged Strategy

It is noteworthy that the educational investment in agriculture can indirectly benefit health. Specifically, IPM Farmer Field School programmes located in malarious areas will inadvertently influence malaria epidemiology if income and living standards are raised (by improving people's access to health care) and if agro-pesticide use is reduced (by lowering the risk of insecticide resistance in malaria vectors). IPM programmes may be complementary to malaria control efforts. A coordinated inter-sectoral planning and implementation of activities could potentially make better use of scarce resources and synergise effects. It is proposed that integration could be taken one step further. A logical adaptation of the IPM Farmer Field School is to make the ecology and control of malaria disease implicit in the IPM curriculum, by purposely involving farmers and other interested actors in the management of malaria in their environment.

This combined strategy, labeled Integrated Pest and Vector Management (IPVM), can be expected to affect malaria disease in four different ways (Figure 2). First, as mentioned above, a reduced use of agro-pesticides, the most consistent outcome of IPM Farmer Field School pro-grammes, will lower the risk of resistance in the vector. Second, experiential learning leads to practical knowledge about the ecology and epidemiology of malaria, which could influence personal protection measures or treatment-seeking behaviour. Third, IPM results in increased income from agriculture, due to increased yield and due to savings in pesticide expenditure [17]. An economic outcome may benefit nutrition, housing conditions and access to health services. Fourth, environmental management by farming communities is expected to suppress mosquito breeding and, consequently, to reduce the period and/or intensity of disease transmission. Critical issues in environmental management are the portion of breeding sites covered, the local landscape and possible increased fitness or survival of the vector at reduced population density. Reduction of nuisance mosquitoes (which is in itself a benefit), could affect bednet use unless this matter is taken up in the FFS curriculum.

This broad range of outcomes implies that the IPVM methodology is not necessarily restricted to situations where prospects for environmental management exist. IPVM could be targeted to address rural poverty, awareness or pesticide overuse, even in areas where environmental management is not an option.

Rice as Starting Point

Synergistic relationships between rice cultivation and vector management have long been known [19], which makes wetland rice a promising starting point for an integrated strategy. Wetland rice can produce large vector populations, though not necessarily of high vectorial capacity. Interruption of vector breeding in leveled fields is often technically feasible through regular drainage [20] or through appropriate management during the fallow period [21]. Considering the flight radius of anophelines, however, field-level management would need to be implemented over a sufficient area to have an effect on vector populations. This requires active participation of large numbers of farmers. In many irrigation situations, water management is insufficiently controlled by individual farmers, although this is potentially improved through the FFS and its socio-political impacts.

In epidemic-prone areas at the margins of malaria transmission, or in areas with strong seasonal malaria, a reduced period or intensity of transmission is expected to cause a temporary decline in malarial disease, because parasitaemia usually results in disease in non-immune people. In parts of Africa with stable holoendemic malaria, a reduced transmission is expected to reduce the risk of severe disease, particularly in infants and young children before they have acquired a certain level of natural immunity [22]. As far as possible, environmental management of malaria needs to be conducted alongside other locally-appropriate control interventions, under an evidence-based Integrated Vector Management (IVM) approach [6]. Ultimately, the impact of community-based activities on local transmission and morbidity of malaria needs to be assessed. This requires locally clustered field school programmes to achieve an appropriate scale, a control and local measurements of transmission and morbidity.

Adapted Curriculum

The IPVM Farmer Field School curriculum has recently been developed for the wetland rice ecosystem in Sri Lanka. The project, involving one of us (HvdB), built on the experience of an existing IPM project. Experiential learning exercises on the health component have been developed to complement, not replace, the existing curriculum on IPM.

The process of curriculum development was mostly in the hands of selected IPM facilitators with technical support from health resource persons. Learning objectives for the new curriculum were based on surveys, which were conducted by the facilitators to study the perceptions and knowledge of rural people about vector-borne diseases, in particular malaria. The developed learning exercises used simple and easily replicable methods, as well as locally available materials. The health component was addressed mainly in the first part of the season, when most anopheline breeding takes place. Different gender roles were noted by the facilitators, women showing most interest

Table 1: Exercises on Mosquito Biology, Ecology and Management which were Added to the Agricultural Topics of the Farmer Field School Curriculum

Exercise	Methods	Purpose
1 Agro-ecosystem analysis	Comprehensive sampling of the crop ecosystem (using soup spoons, visual counts, plant measurements, etc.) and visual presentation and analysis.	To monitor the agro-ecosystem and make context-specific decisions on necessary action related to crop production and human health.
2 Mosquito breeding habitat	Dipper sampling in, and characterization of, various aquatic habitats of mosquito genera.	To study where different mosquito genera breed.
3 Adult mosquito sampling	Collecting adult mosquitoes at different times and habitats and identify major genera, i.e., using home-made aspirators.	To monitor potential disease vectors and their activity.
4 Mosquito lifecycle	Rearing of young larvae in water jar covered with mesh.	To understand the relation between maggot, pupae and adult, and the development time.
5 Mosquito identification	Observing larval behaviour and adult characteristics.	To distinguish *Anopheles*, *Aedes* and *Culex* in the larval and adult stage.
6 Predation	Exposing larvae or pupae to a range of arthropods inside jars.	To understand the role of predators in controlling mosquito developmental stages.
7 Analogy on disease cycle	Role play on the cycle of the parasite through human and mosquito hosts.	To understand the role of the vector and the human reservoir.
8 Agricultural methods to suppress mosquito breeding	Alternate wet-dry irrigation of study field plots; land levelling at planting.	To study how farmer practices influence mosquito breeding and crop development.
9 Source reduction	Farmer action to drain or fill water bodies, including in the peri-domestic environment.	To practice measures to contain vector breeding.
10 Mapping	Drawing map of village environment with water bodies, crops, houses, etc.	To facilitate planning for coordinated action on environmental management.

in the health component and men in the agricultural component. Preliminary observations in Sri Lanka suggest that farmers can be motivated and educated to play an active and competent role in vector management. Similar curricula could be included in formal school education in rural areas.

Details of the learning exercises are given in Table 1. Sampling of mosquito developmental stages and aquatic predators was incorporated within the weekly exercise of agro-ecosystem analysis. The exercise was initiated well before planting and continued as long as standing water was available in the field; post-harvest larval breeding had not been identified as an important issue. Farmers learned to recognize the larvae and adults of the three main mosquito genera, *Anopheles*, *Culex* and *Aedes*, using behavioural and taxonomic clues, to study mosquito-breeding habitat, and to monitor adult mosquitoes. Mosquito life cycles and mosquito predators were studied by daily observations inside transparent containers. Land leveling and alternate wet-dry irrigation were implemented in the study plots to manage mosquitoes, and farmers learned to practice source reduction, through filling, draining or manipulating water bodies in their environment. This involved planning, mapping and action by the group of participating farmers. The disease cycle of malaria, a topic unsuitable for practical learning, was addressed through a role-play, whereby farmers were assigned roles of human hosts, vector and parasite stages, and whereby the process of transmission was performed.

Conclusion

As managers of their rural environment, farmers have a role to play in malaria control. An approach aiming to empower and organize farmers to take initiative is presented. The IPVM Farmer Field School connects the health component to agricultural productivity, which broadens the institutional basis of malaria control and provides an economic incentive mechanism necessary to motivate people into action. Adaptation of the approach to other agro-ecosystems with associated vector breeding (e.g., irrigated vegetables, cotton, ridge crops) requires further study. The approach has potential to raise living standards of the rural poor above a threshold level at which people have the means to combat malaria. As educational investment, the IPVM Farmer Field School is expected to cause a lasting and profound change in people and in their relationship with the environment. Costs of up-scaling field school activities do not necessarily come from projects or public health budgets, but institutional ownership and support could potentially be shared by sectors of health, agriculture, education, irrigation and environment. Hence, a process for institutional learning and reform needs to be initiated.

Acknowledgements

The late Felix P. Amerasinghe is remembered for his inspiration and great efforts that helped develop the IPVM approach. The authors are indebted to all those who are or have been involved in the Sri Lankan project, from the Department of Agriculture, Anti-Malaria Campaign, Mahaweli Authority, and FAO, for sharing in their experience. Particularly acknowledged are Laxman Amarasinghe, A.A. George, D.M. Gunawardena, N.B. Munasingha, Nalin Munasinghe, and Hector Senerath.

(Henk van den Berg (Corresponding Author), Laboratory of Entomology, Wageningen University and Research Centre, Wageningen, The Netherlands. The author can be reached at henk.vandenberg@wur.nl;

Bart GJ Knols is with Laboratory of Entomology, Wageningen University and Research Centre, Wageningen, The Netherlands and also with International Atomic Energy Agency (IAEA), Agency's Laboratories Seibersdorf, Austria. The author can be reached at b.knols@iaea.org).

References

1. Klinkenberg E, McCall PJ, Hastings IA, Wilson MD, Amerasinghe FP, Donnelly MJ: Malaria and irrigated crops, Accra, Ghana. *Emerg Infect Dis* 2005, 11:1290-1293.
2. Wang SJ, Lengeler C, Smith TA, Vounatsou P, Diadie DA, Pritroipa X, Convelbo N, Kientga M, Tanner M: Rapid urban malaria appraisal (RUMA) I: Epidemiology of urban malaria in Ouagadougou. *Malar J* 2005, 4:43.
3. Georghiou GP: The effect of agrochemicals on vector populations. *Pesticide Resistance in Arthropods, RT Roush & BE Tabashnik* 1990:183-202.
4. Diabate A, Baldet T, Chandre F, Akogbeto M, Guiguemde TR, Darriet F, Brengues C, Guillet P, Hemingway J, Small GJ, Hougard JM: The role of agricultural use of insecticides in resistance to pyre-throids in *Anopheles gambiae s.l.* in Burkina Faso. *Am J Trop Med Hyg* 2002, 67:617-622.
5. Darriet FGP, N'Guessan R, Doannio JMC, Koffi A, Konan LY, Carnev-ale P: Impact de la résistance d' *Anopheles gambiae s.s.* méthrine et àine sur l'efficacité des moustiquaires impregnées. *Méde Tropl* 1998, 58:349-354.

6. WHO: Global strategic framework for Integrated Vector Management. Geneva: WHO; 2004.

7. Ghebreyesus TA, Witten KH, Getachew A, O'Neill K, Bosman A, Teklehaimanot A: Community-based malaria control in Tigray, northern Ethiopia. *Parassitologia* 1999, 41:367-371.

8. Kidane G, Morrow RH: Teaching mothers to provide home treatment of malaria in Tigray, Ethiopia: A randomised trial. *Lancet* 2000, 356:550-555.

9. Armstrong-Schellenberg JRM, Abdulla S, Nathan R, Mukasa O, March-ant TJ, Kikumbih N, Mushi AK, Mponda H, Minja H, Mshinda H, Tanner M, Lengeler C: Effect of large-scale social marketing of insecticide-treated nets on child survival in rural Tanzania. *Lancet* 2001, 340:1241-1247.

10. Service MW: Community participation in vector-borne disease control. *Ann Trop Med Parasitol* 1993, 87:223-234.

11. Sharma RC, Gautam AS, Bhatt RM, Gupta DK, Sharma VP: The Kheda malaria project: the case for environmental control. *Health Policy Plan* 1991, 6:262-270.

12. Lindsay SW, Egwang TG, Kabuye F, Mutambo T, Matwale GK: Community-based environmental management program for malaria control in Kampala and Jinja, Uganda. Final Report. *Washington: Environmental Health Project* 2004.

13. Keiser J, Singer BH, Utzinger J: Reducing the burden of malaria in different eco-epidemiological settings with environmental management: a systematic review. *Lancet Infect Dis* 2005, 5: 695-708.

14. Pretty JN: Participatory learning for sustainable agriculture. *World Dev* 1995, 23:1247-1263.

15. UN-Millenium-Project: Halving Hunger: It can be done. *Task Force on Hunger* 2005:123.

16. Braun A, Jiggins J, Röling N, van den Berg H, Snijders P: A global survey and review of Farmer Field School experiences. Nairobi: International Livestock Research Institute; 2006.

17. van den Berg H: IPM Farmer Field Schools: A synthesis of 25 impact evaluations. Rome: Global IPM Facility; 2004.

18. Pontius JC, Dilts DR, Bartlett A: Ten years of IPM training in Asia: From Farmer Field School to community IPM. Bangkok: FAO; 2002.

19. Mather TH, That TT: Environmental management for vector control in rice fields. FAO Irrigation and Drainage Papers 41. Rome: FAO; 1984.

20. Keiser J, Utzinger J, Singer BH: The potential of intermittent irrigation for increasing rice yields, lowering water consumption, reducing methane emissions, and controlling malaria in African rice fields. *J Am Mosq Control Assoc* 2002, 18:329-340.

21. Klinkenberg E, Takken W, Huibers F, Touré YT: The phenology of malaria mosquitoes in irrigated rice fields in Mali. *Acta Trop* 2003, 85:71-82.

22. Smith TA, Leuenberger R, Lengeler C: Child mortality and malaria transmission intensity in Africa. *Trends Parasitol* 2001, 17:145-149.

Index

A

Accessibility, 4, 12, 35, 39, 44, 58, 60, 94, 95, 101, 189, 203
Accreditation, 83, 88, 95
Advocacy, 62, 65, 66, 88, 95
Affordability, 185, 186, 188, 203
Agro-Pesticide, 216-218
Algorithmic, 49
Allopathic, 9, 198, 200, 203
ArcObjects, 56
Articulated, 166, 168
Atmosphere, 146, 147

B

Beneficiaries, 23, 123
Biennially, 7
Biodiversity, 10

C

Cardiovascular/Respiratory, 162
Catastrophic, 5, 16, 20, 24, 121, 122, 181, 199, 200, 202
Charitable, 21, 199-202
Chronic, 26-29, 31, 33-35, 139, 140, 142, 143, 156, 204, 209
Chunk, 3
Client-Server, 41
Clinical, 7, 28, 32, 33, 35, 78, 80, 83, 87, 89-91, 97, 102, 148, 149, 202, 203
Cluster, 197-202
Collaborative, 19, 27, 29-31, 35, 58, 60, 108, 156, 196
Commuting, 153
Companion, 85, 176
Competitive, 66
Compounded, 5, 74
Comprehensive, 102, 158, 197, 202
Constraints, 4, 5, 12, 84, 154, 186, 196
Conversely, 22, 46
Coordinated, 77, 140, 196, 197, 217, 218
Counterparts, 17, 41, 170
Criteria, 38, 46, 47, 133, 208
Curriculum, 75, 94, 96, 218, 219
Cylinders, 202

D

Database, 27, 34, 42, 54-56, 178, 198, 209
Decentralised, 75
Dengue, 5, 6
Deplorable, 5
Diabetes, 27-31, 33-35
Diarrhea, 140, 197
Diet, 164, 166
Diligently, 66
Disparities, 28, 30, 31, 35, 57, 173, 179
Dissemination, 40, 61-64, 66-68
Distressed, 157, 175
Distribution, 8, 37, 58, 129, 131, 178, 179, 213

Diversification, 192
Domestic, 99, 131
Dominating, 151
Drug, 10, 126, 157

E

Electronic, 13, 27, 28, 30, 35, 65-67, 100, 138, 148
Empowerment, 214, 215, 217
Entire, 31, 43, 89, 133, 141, 147, 183, 198
Ethnography, 8
Ethnomedicine, 9, 11
Exacerbating, 5
Expanded, 13, 24, 42, 59, 63, 79, 115
Expectancy, 156

F

Federal, 13, 36, 38, 62, 67, 68, 70, 83, 85, 87, 88, 90, 91, 97-99, 101, 102, 104, 106, 108, 155, 156
Federally, 31, 85
Fevers, 140
Four-Dimensional, 152
Frontier, 18, 82, 85-88, 93-98, 100-102, 104-106, 113

G

Genetics, 155, 164, 166

H

Hasty Retreat, 141
Healing, 8-11, 14, 136
Homeostasis, 196
Homicides, 88
Homogeneous, 23, 197
Hospitalization, 5, 19, 181, 191

I

Ideology, 78
Immunization, 6, 7, 14, 59, 122, 179
Indicators, 27-29, 88, 152, 153, 155-158, 161-164, 166, 170, 172-175
Indigenous, 10, 139, 142
Infant, 5, 156, 204, 209, 219
Infrastructure, 11-13, 17, 31, 41, 57, 63, 68, 84, 89, 94, 98, 100, 102, 107, 131, 133, 140, 155, 194, 196-198, 200, 201, 203
Initial, 44, 46, 78, 100, 134, 135, 204, 207, 208
Injury, 87-89, 112
Inpatient, 44, 107, 118, 122, 127, 129, 179
Insecticides, 214, 222
Insufficient, 84, 178
Insurers, 83, 115, 122, 126-128
Integrated, 12, 29, 43, 58, 84, 86, 91, 103, 104, 173, 214, 216-219, 223
Interdisciplinary, 28, 35, 90, 92, 174, 197, 214
Intermediaries, 21, 65, 185
Interoperable, 94, 100, 101, 103
Investigate, 80, 99, 151
Iteratively, 197

J

Jurisdictional, 65

L

Licensure, 95, 112
Logistics, 139, 140, 144, 179

M

Macroeconomics, 21
Maternity, 44, 46, 53, 54, 56, 180, 191

Metaphors, 42
Metropolitan, 13, 43, 44, 53, 54
Minimal, 27, 34, 41, 98, 193
Minorities, 17, 70
Misallocated, 180
Mixture, 125, 164
Mobilization, 22, 215
Monetary, 179, 188, 193, 199-202, 207
Monitoring, 8, 9, 14, 34, 38, 100-102, 181
Morbidity, 178, 180, 204, 209, 219
Mortality, 5, 8, 156, 178, 204, 209, 224
Multi-Disciplinary, 87

N

Nurse-Translator, 140-143

O

Occurrence, 89, 181
Ophthalmology, 132
Organism, 196, 217
Outpatient, 107, 122, 127, 179, 180
Oversight, 87, 95, 96, 99
Overwhelming, 12, 177
Oxygen, 202, 203

P

Paramedic, 55
Participation, 21, 22, 24, 40, 80, 90, 147, 162, 163, 164, 188, 214, 215, 219, 223
Peripherally, 83
Planthoppers, 217
Plethora, 9, 10
Polygons, 53
Predominantly, 178, 181
Premiums, 19, 23, 182, 184, 187, 188
Problematic, 96, 103
Progressively, 182
Prompt, 28, 122
Provincial, 38, 44, 45, 60, 156, 169
Provisionary, 187

Q

Quantifying, 19

R

Reallocations, 43, 44
Recommendations, 62, 64, 85-93, 95, 97, 100, 104, 107, 108
Reimbursement, 32, 91, 96-99, 107, 119, 125, 130
Reliable, 65, 99

S

Scheme, 5, 19-25, 116, 118-123, 128, 183, 185-187, 191-194
Shortfall, 180
Socioeconomic, 4, 19, 23, 24, 176
Sonography, 100, 199-202
Sparse, 187
Spatial, 39, 50, 52, 56-59, 152
Spectacular, 116
Spectrum, 102, 119, 214
Stabilization, 85, 89, 169
Standardized, 27, 31, 89, 96
Stockpiling, 94
Streamlining, 39
Sub-Optimal, 18
Substantially, 20, 63, 123, 161
Superfluous, 64
Superimposed, 140

Surmounted, 136
Surveillance, 8, 57, 90, 100, 102, 103
Sustainability, 13, 35, 153, 164, 168, 170-172, 188, 207, 214, 215
Synthesis, 63, 223

T

Telemedicine, 3, 13, 15, 94, 100, 101, 103, 131-137
Territorial, 95, 156
Timeframes, 63
Toolkits, 90
Township, 120, 121, 124
Trachoma, 140, 142
Transitioned, 118
Translated, 64
Trauma, 44, 46, 53, 54, 56, 60, 85-89, 91, 95, 99-101, 103-105, 107-111
Triage, 87, 89-91, 97, 138, 140-143, 146, 147
Triennially, 7

U

Underutilization, 182
Unforeseen, 199, 200
Unique, 17, 30, 84, 89, 93, 97, 107, 184, 186

V

Vaccine, 7, 14, 203
Vector, 59, 214, 217-219, 221-223
Verbal, 65
Visualize, 46, 53
Voluntary, 9, 21, 32, 120, 122
Vulnerability, 6, 17

Z

Zootherapy, 11